The Owl at the Window

Carl Gorham created the animated show *Stressed Eric* for BBC2 and adapted the best-selling *Meg and Mog* children's books for ITV.

He has also written sketches, monologues and sitcoms for both radio and television including *The Gorham and Swift Show* (BBC Radio 2), *The Very Old Pretenders* (BBC Radio 4) and, most recently, a new sitcom pilot *Martin* for ITV starring Alan Davies.

He has won numerous awards including two British Animation Awards and an Indie, and he is a British Comedy Award and Bafta nominee.

He lives in North Norfolk with his daughter.

CARL GORHAM

The Owl at the Window

A memoir of loss and hope

CORONET

First published in Great Britain in 2017 by Coronet
An Imprint of Hodder & Stoughton
An Hachette UK company

This paperback edition published in 2018

1

Copyright © Carl Gorham 2017

A CIP catalogue record for this title is available from the British Library

B format ISBN 9781473642331

Typeset in 10.75/15.25pt Plantin Light by
Palimpsest Book Production Limited, Falkirk, Stirlingshire

Printed and bound in Great Britain by Clays Ltd, St Ives plc

Hodder & Stoughton policy is to use papers that are natural, renewable
and recyclable products and made from wood grown in sustainable
forests. The logging and manufacturing processes are expected to
conform to the environmental regulations of the country of origin.

Hodder & Stoughton Ltd
Carmelite House
50 Victoria Embankment
London EC4Y 0DZ

www.hodder.co.uk

For Vikki and Romy.

I

BACK IN TIME

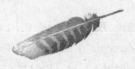

I am eight years old and it's the school holidays. I'm looking out of the lounge window at the road which curls past and spins off into the distance: the clean pavement, the long front gardens that lead to the brick-built houses with sloping tiled roofs, each three storeys high in blocks of four. New modern houses with the promise of a new modern life.

I can see other children walking down the road past the houses, off to the park or the shops. The boys are play-fighting, trying to trip each other up. The girls let out huge exaggerated laughs and outbursts of mock horror as they exchange gossip. Their noise punctures the air for there are few other sounds. There's no great industry and little traffic on the roads, just the purring of a light breeze and the odd exclamation from the cattle market near the station; it's the soundtrack of a small Sussex town in the early 1970s.

I'm watching all of this but I'm quite happy, for I am a loner. A contented, fulfilled, loner. I can disappear for days to my bedroom and just hang out there on my own. Not that I don't have any friends, I do – Wal, Pooley, Lil. But I often don't feel the need to see them. I'm fine by myself.

Particularly today. Because today I am a longbowman from Agincourt. I have on a suede jacket with the arms cut off that I got from Auntie Rae. This forms a medieval jerkin and is worn over an old white school shirt that has been ripped about. I have also borrowed some tights and have made a longbow from a tree at the bottom of my garden. I'm still working on the shoes and I have in mind some sort of leather boots, soft ankle-high moccasins maybe, or crude bindings made from animal hide fastened with hemp. At the moment I'm making do with socks.

Today I'm a bowman, but tomorrow I might be a redcoat from 1815 or Alfred the Great or an eighteenth-century French cuirassier or a bomber pilot from 1945. I like to dress up as historical characters. I've always liked it. Other boys might build small fires or do wheelies or climb trees. Each day I come down to breakfast dressed as someone from the past, though recently I have had to abandon being Nelson because the tomato ketchup I put on to his frilly shirt has started to smell.

I have a large hollow stool whose seat opens up, and inside I store the shirts, coats, lengths of material, belts, ornaments and weapons that make up my historical ward-

2

robe. I have borrowed them from relatives and friends and picked up stuff from jumble sales and school fairs. My mum once bid in an auction for an eighteenth-century back-woodsman's pistol but could only go to seven pounds: any more, and it would have eaten into the family holiday budget.

I like to dress up as these different people and be them all day. I call it 'thinks'. I'm happy when I'm doing 'thinks'. I don't need anyone else to join in. In fact, I don't want anyone to join in. They'd say the wrong thing, do the wrong thing. They'd laugh.

But to me it's serious. I don't just dress as these characters: I become them. I am no longer myself. I am no longer eight years old in a middle-class town near Brighton. When I put on these special clothes I'm back there, in time, in history. I build mantraps and fight opponents. I go on secret missions. I'm taken prisoner and escape. I give chase. I scheme. I plot. I build dens and go to sleep wrapped in my cloak.

I build Hampton Court or Agincourt or the inside of a Lancaster bomber in the living room, turning up the furniture, making houses out of the sofa cushions and emptying the airing cupboard to use sheets fastened with clothes pegs as walls. I carve utensils from tree branches in the garden and eat food from a rough old breadboard I've taken from the kitchen.

And once I've built these places I stay there, live there, become part of that life.

My family is accepting. When I come down to breakfast in the morning, my father lowers his paper and asks, 'Who are you today?'

I reply, 'A longbowman from Agincourt.'

He says, 'Oh, good,' then continues as if I've just told him that the weather is going to be sunny or England has beaten the West Indies at cricket.

He's totally genuine though. When he says, 'Good,' he means it. In his eyes my 'thinks' are creative, and anything creative is to be applauded. The only thing he fears me becoming is an accountant or a lawyer in life – he's told me that. He'd rather I ran away and joined the circus.

My father is creative too. He writes poetry and paints and on Saturday mornings he often makes me objects I can use when I'm having 'thinks'. He has made me a magnificent papier-mâché mace from the Middle Ages and a two-handed sword out of cardboard – it has an intricate handle inlaid with jewels (buttons). He is planning to make me a shield but we don't quite have enough cardboard – he wants to stick several layers together because he says it has to be strong enough to withstand the blow from an axe.

My mother is just as supportive. For months now she has been making me a suit of chain mail. She has managed to get a pattern from a local theatre group who have just done a production of Saint Joan. *The thread she uses is thick, like rope, and she weaves it together in a complex cross-stitch using giant knitting needles; the idea is to spray it silver afterwards so it looks like metal.*

She has been labouring long and hard for nearly six months, late at night, but she hasn't shown me anything yet. Until now.

'Here it is,' she says. She holds up a chain-mail hood – the result of her hours and hours of hard graft. The stitching is immaculate, the texture perfect, and it looks as if it could be on display in the Tower of London even though it has yet to be coloured. She smiles as she holds it out. 'There,' she says proudly. 'What do you think?'

I take it from her and hold it up to the light. Then I look at her hands, red and gnarled from their labours, and her bright, sweet, optimistic face, alive with expectation. 'Where's the rest of it?' I say.

It's a Saturday morning in the same year. It's hot, especially in the shopping arcade where I'm standing, which is packed with people. It's a small arcade, not particularly spectacular or glamorous, not one of those show-off Victorian arcades you get in London. It's scruffy, provincial, like the rest of Brighton before it became bohemian and hip.

I'm standing outside Gamley's, the biggest toy shop in the town, and I'm wearing khaki shorts and a T-shirt with horizontal stripes. I'm alone and I'm clutching an Airfix model kit of King Charles I. What's more, I'm holding it in front of my crotch and I'm crying.

My English Civil War 'thinks' have been particularly

strong over the last few months and have dominated my every waking hour. I've got some books on the Battle of Naseby from the library, I've been to see the film Cromwell, starring Richard Harris, and my mum has written off on my behalf to see if I might become a very junior member of the Sealed Knot Society.

I've been drawn instinctively to the Roundhead side, partly because the Ladybird book on Cromwell that I'm basing most of my research on seems to describe him, with the exception of what happens in Ireland, as a hero, and partly because Mum and Dad are suspicious of the royal family and vote Labour.

So I have organised a complete parliamentarian officer's outfit – the suede jacket from Auntie Rae that was my Agincourt bowman's jerkin now recut to make a seventeenth-century cavalryman's coat, accompanied by some long boots from a church jumble sale, which are the right height, if a little bit girly, and a cummerbund made out of some old curtain material, which is tied around my waist.

I have paraded around the house and galloped through the hallway wearing the outfit. I have restaged all the battles – Naseby, Marston Moor. I have even made speeches to my troops, standing on an old tea chest at the bottom of the garden. I have lived, breathed and slept the life of a Roundhead.

The trouble is, I'm starting to tire of it now – the dull, conformist colours of the clothes, the respectful, disciplined *living, the lack of laughter (apparently Roundheads didn't even smile much). In fact, truth be told, I've found myself wondering what it would be like to be a Royalist – daring and wild, colourful and free. Galloping up and down the garden, waving my hat in the air and laughing uproariously.*

So I decide to switch sides.

Making a Royalist outfit, though, is not easy: my house is a bit short on fine silks, and achieving a decent ruff around the neck is well-nigh impossible – the closest I get is a forlorn attempt to reshape some cake doilies with a pair of nail scissors. I persist, I experiment, I even try origami but, try as I might, I can't get anything like the look I want. I feel stuck. No costume, no possibility of a costume. Yet my new enthusiasm for being a Royalist just seems to grow.

I then discover that the model-maker Airfix includes Charles I in their historical figures series. The figures are seven inches high, composed of forty or fifty parts, which you put together, then glue onto a plinth.

Immediately I become fixated on getting one, all the enthusiasm for the failed outfit now redirected towards a plastic figure the size of a small garden gnome.

I dream of painting the various sections, gluing them together, then sitting the finished model proudly and elegantly on the little desk next to my bed, along with my Ladybird book on Charles I and maybe a hat with a feather on it. I foresee a whole Royalist display in that corner of my bedroom, with the Airfix figure as the centrepiece. My desire to get one becomes all-consuming. It's an obsession that haunts my every waking hour.

None of the local shops seems to have a Charles I. They can supply a Richard I, they can supply several Napoleons and even an Anne Boleyn, but no Charles.

We ring up places further afield. We ask friends and relatives. We look in newspapers and magazines. Finally we track down a batch of Charles's in Gamley's, the toy store in Brighton, a short train ride away.

Brighton to me is all about dreams and great moments. Excitement and fun. Always has been. My strongest childhood memories are bound up with the place, among its Regency streets and handsome squares; on the boisterous colourful pier; near the beautiful, barmy Prince Regent's Palace; in the crumbling old football stadium with its noise and smell of cheap hotdogs.

Brighton is where I have my first kiss, go to my first live gig, and drink too much alcohol for the first time while dancing the night away. Brighton is my inspiration, my gateway, my escape, my first glimpse into another more exciting world. Brighton is where it all starts.

We come out of the station and follow the main road that falls away to the sea, a walk of faded chip shops and Victorian bars, an elegant handrail stitching them together as it accompanies you down the hill. When we get to the clock tower we turn right, up a small incline towards the main body of the shops, towards the arcade.

It's a walk of colour, of vivid smells. A walk of tingling anticipation.

When we get to the door of the shop my mum and dad give me the money to buy the figure, then arrange to meet me afterwards – they are popping next door to C & A. I don't wait to watch them turn and disappear before I spin round and speed inside.

It is sitting there in a shiny rectangular box, with the Airfix logo and a full-scale picture of the contents. It is Charles I and it is the only one left.

Quickly I pick it up. I shiver as I lift it: it's every bit as beautiful as I imagined. I hold it in my hand, disbelieving, joyous and fulfilled. And then I become aware of something else, another reason why I'm shivering.

I want to go to the loo. Quite badly.

Clearly I've been focusing so intently on this moment that everything else has been ignored. All other thoughts, sensations, ambitions have been shelved, shut down in my single-minded obsessive quest, including the usual signals that it's time to empty my bladder.

Still, no matter – a quick trip to the loo, then I can nip back and make the purchase. I put the box down carefully, making sure it's as far out of sight on the shelf as possible. Then I look round . . .

And see another boy, not much older than me, looking along the same shelf.

He is working his way unerringly towards me, past a couple of Richard Is, past Henry VIII, past Julius Caesar.

9

He picks up each in turn, looks at it for a minute, then replaces it on the shelf. He's going to take King Charles from me. I know it.

I reach back in, pick up the box and head for the till, the need for the loo so acute now that I feel the occasional sharp pain around my midriff and I'm conscious of taking small steps. There is a queue. I brace myself, determined. I've got this far and I'm not going to give in. Two people ahead of me. Just two. I can manage that. Even if the sharp pain around my midriff is coming more frequently.

The woman operating the till is speaking to the person at the front of the queue. 'You got much shopping to do?'

'Not really, just Marks, then Habitat.'

'Oooh, you should see some of the stuff they've got in there. So lovely. How's Bob?'

Oh no. They're friends! Please hurry up. Please.

The pain in my midriff is spreading. I can feel a twinge in my back now too. A wave of panic grips me. I feel trapped. There is no way out. I look around – my rival is still loitering by the Airfix models, a clear and present danger. My breathing gets shallower. I look down at my fingers, which clutch Charles I so tightly that the knuckles are a bloodless white. I can feel a drop of sweat snaking down my back inside my T-shirt.

When I look up again the chatty woman is leaving. It's okay. Everything is going to be okay, I tell myself. We all shuffle up one, towards the till. As we do, I'm conscious of having to tighten my groin muscles even more. They can't go any further.

'That'll be eight pound fifty,' says the lady behind the counter.

That's good. Straight to the point. And, even better, the customer in front of me is a man. A man is less likely to do friendly chatting. Plus, he's only got one thing – a chemistry set. He's giving it to the till lady now. And he's got the money too.

Yes! Thank you, Man-with-a-chemistry-set.

The till lady suddenly stops. 'Oh, run out of bags. Hang on.' She looks up. 'Maureen?'

Maureen, who is stacking shelves on the other side of the room, walks slowly towards her.

HURRY UP MAUREEN OR I'M GOING TO WET MYSELF.

I wince. The pain is now so severe that I have to stoop and cross one leg in front of the other.

'Are you all right?' asks Maureen.

'Yes,' I croak. 'I'm—'

I start to pee on the floor.

At first it's just a few drops. Then a few more. And then a few more.

Before long it's a stream and a little dark patch appears on the light blue carpet at my feet, like a cloud on a previously perfect day.

'Don't worry, love,' says Maureen, cheerfully. 'I've seen worse.'

I move to one side in the vain hope that by shifting my position I might be able to get hold of my bladder again *but it doesn't work. All it means is that another cloud appears next to the one that has already formed. I move again and again with a similar result. Soon there is a number of little clouds at my feet, and all I can do is try to stand on them in a desperate attempt to cover them up.*

'*Really, don't worry,*' *says Maureen, kindly.* '*It can be cleaned.*'

The carpet is now a patchwork of dark clouds and I'm hopping around on them from foot to foot as if I'm involved in a bizarre game of Twister. Other people are starting to stare at me, the strange, sad, dancing child with tears in his eyes and a sizeable wet patch on his shorts, but I won't let go of the Airfix model. I won't let it go. I WON'T LET IT GO. IT'S MINE. I hold it out of danger, out of harm's way, at the end of my outstretched arm till my bladder is empty and the light carpet has become a dark sky and the people who were watching have lost interest and turned away.

Needless to say, when my mother and father finally come to collect me from the shop, I'm already standing outside, in the street, as far away from the scene of my crime as possible.

But as we walk back to the station, with their consoling arms around me and their comforting words in my ears, it dawns on me that this was no disaster: my mission has been accomplished. I have indeed bought the very last model of King Charles I, which I am now holding diplomatically in a horizontal position to cover the wet patch on my crotch.

And though I'm still crying, still shaking and still ashamed, inside I'm triumphant.

A container houses the Airfix model of Charles I and the chain-mail hood. It also holds an old copy of the Mid Sussex Times *with a picture of me dressed as Sherlock Holmes's assistant in a school play, a Subbuteo pitch and a book I won as an English prize at secondary school. I find that container in the first few frantic days after I return from Hong Kong as I'm looking for a different box, the one that has the family documents, the birth and marriage certificates, the stuff you need when someone dies.*

Several similar boxes are piled high in the bottom of the wardrobe. They are plastic and rectangular with tops that clip on. They get rough treatment, these boxes, being moved around, stacked and bumped. We don't have much storage space in our house. The boxes have scratches but they work. They do the job. They look after the past.

In the mad scramble to find the documents, I pull out all these boxes, rip the lids off and there they are, mementoes of a young life, a little dusty, smaller than I remember them, smelling of the seventies and the hard plastic of an airless container that's rarely opened.

I find myself thinking of the eight-year-old boy who wore the chain-mail and peed in a toy shop just so he wouldn't lose his dream. I think of his naivety, his self-absorption, his youthful insensitivity. I see his delight, his obsessiveness.

So free. So oblivious.

I think of the life ahead, its unexpected twists and turns, and the darkness that will gather. I think of him and how ill-equipped he is to face it all. And I want to warn him.

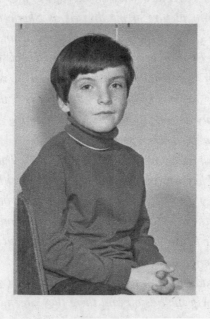

A STRANGE KIND OF SHOPPING

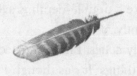

'Would you like a double-depth grave?'

It's not a question you expect to hear. Not now, not while you're in your early forties with a six-year-old child. The words echo around the room, elusive and far away. As if they're meant for someone else.

'Mr Gorham?' The funeral director looks at me. She is wearing a black business suit that seems a bit too tight for her. It strains under the armpits and is creased at the front where a single button holds the jacket shut. Whenever she speaks, she leans forward and does a comforting little smile at the end of each sentence, but the smiles are so frequent that, after a while, they rather lose their impact. She is seated at a large table opposite Vikki's father, mother, sister and me and has various brochures in front of her containing pictures of coffins, bunches of flowers and funeral cars. The office that surrounds her is light and airy. The wallpaper is gentle, nondescript, and there are few signs that this is an undertakers, save for a small bunch of flowers in a vase. With her brochures and her professionally friendly manner she could be selling me a bathroom.

'Would you like a double-depth grave? Mr Gorham?' She smiles patiently at me.

My whole body aches. I'm exhausted by the effort of keeping up with things. It's as though I've been running a race in which I've been lapped over and over again. My limbs are heavy, my mouth is dry. I'm reeling from it all, my head spinning, my thoughts hanging.

My wife is dead. She has actually died. And this is yet another reminder.

I can't believe it. Can't process it. I can't actually work with the information.

Wait. Stop everything. A minute, please.

She is *dead*.

She is dead and I am still with those words. That moment. Everything else is just rushing past.

She is dead.

She was here just now and she was alive.

How can she suddenly be dead? People in history are dead. Old people are dead. Grandparents are dead. Other people are dead. Not people like me. Not this person. The person I was married to. Had a child with. Not the person who was standing next to me. Chatting. Laughing. Being.

'Er . . . Double . . . er . . . ?'

'Depth. For both of you,' she says.

'But it's my wife who's . . .'

'Of course, but we have to look ahead. It's difficult to change it once it's dug.' She does that professional smile again.

I stumble on: 'In that case we'd better . . . er . . . double . . . er . . .'

But she is already looking down at her notepad and writing the answer. 'Depth,' she mouths, as she writes the word. She looks up again. 'Now, obviously we'll have to wait till the coffin comes back from Hong Kong to check it. It might well be that it's been damaged in transit – that often happens. It might be absolutely fine, of course, in which case we won't need to have a replacement, but in the meantime, I don't know if you want to have a look – consider other options . . . Just in case.'

She turns one of the brochures on the pile towards us and flips through the pages with practised fingers.

Inside are pictures of coffins – some made of oak, others made of elm, several that are mixes of various woods. They are in a bizarre variety of styles too, called things like 'Classic' and 'Victorian' and 'Gothic'.

'This might give you some ideas,' she says.

She flips the page again. This time it is coffin handles.

Twirly ones, swirly ones. Others with little knots in. Some that look like they belong in Middle Earth. A few that are straight and military. The odd minimalist one.

Several that dip in the middle and curve out at the ends. Brass ones, silver ones, iron ones, steel ones.

'It would probably be something plain,' I say, bewildered.

The other family members nod their assent.

She writes something else on her notepad, then looks up again. 'So, we'll wait and see on that. Now, if you wouldn't mind telling me how much your wife weighed?'

'Er . . .'

'Pall bearers,' she says by way of explanation.

My wife is a weight now. An issue. A practical problem. Just a body. Not a person. A weight. My head spins once more. Another punch. A boxer on the ropes when the blows are raining in. Every second. Every sentence.

'Right . . . Er . . . nine stone.'

'That should be fine,' she says, smiling again.

She flicks through several more brochures, then one showing hearses. It contains a range of vehicles, including a horse-drawn option, which would suit an East End gangster. For a mad moment, I'm tempted to go for the horse; it looks fabulous.

'I think probably just the standard hearse,' I say, looking at the family, who again nod in agreement. She adds it to her list, alongside the numbers of pall bearers, the coffin, its associated furniture, and the words 'double-depth'.

It continues in this vein, the surreal shopping trip we're on, as we order the various elements we need for the special, odd, nightmarish day we're duty-bound to organise. There's the question of flowers, details of who is to collect charitable donations, even the colours of the carnations the pall bearers will wear. We decide against the self-watering tree of remembrance. We also decide we don't want to do a deal for a gravestone in polished granite from China – even though we could have got it at a reduced price because we're booking the funeral at the same time.

As the business is finally concluded, we stand up and so does she. Hands are shaken, heads nodded, and she gives out one more of her gentle smiles.

The light is now filtering through the window into her office, illuminating the glossy pile of brochures on the table. For a second, as they shine and glow, they seem almost glamorous. It is a bright day. A beautiful day. But not for everyone.

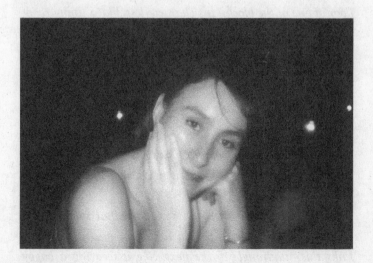

3

JOY DIVISION AND DELACROIX

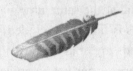

It is a Saturday night in Holywell Quad at Hertford College, Oxford, a cobbled square surrounded by concrete blocks on three sides. Students file out of the small hall on the ground floor of one of the blocks. It's characterless, like a living room in an old people's home, with strip lighting and tatty armchairs pushed back against the wall. At one end of the hall a DJ is dismantling a disco with a cumbersome deck and large unwieldy speakers. It is 1983 – long before they learned how to make them smaller.

The students fill the quad with laughter as they trickle out. Some remain in groups. Others stumble off in different directions, trying to find their way back to their room. Or someone else's.

Vikki – she prefers this quirky individual spelling – is standing opposite me in the narrow stone passageway that links this quadrangle to the next. She is wearing a baggy red silk top and white jeans that show off her figure. She is above average height and has short dark hair and pale skin. She also has beautiful dark eyes. They are what you notice. That, and the cool, distant, exotic air that hangs around her, which I have found irresistible ever since I saw her cool, distant, exotic Czech surname on the college noticeboard.

Vikki and I have been watching each other off and on all evening. We have been with the same large group of friends and there have been a lot of stares but no conversation. Once we ended up in a four, dancing close to each other. Another time I saw her looking at me and glanced back but she immediately turned away.

We've been circling each other for a while now. She is in the year above me – you get to know who everyone is in a small college like ours – and we pass each other from time to time, walking to lectures or climbing the stairs leading to the dining room or queuing to use one of the machines in the launderette.

But now it is just the two of us. For the first time. The others seem to have melted away. We stare at each other. Then, in an effort to look cool, I pull out a packet of cigarettes and offer her one. She takes it and I fumble in my pocket for matches. I strike one and light her cigarette. She doesn't say a word, just stares back at me with those eyes.

I take another cigarette from the packet and put it into my mouth. I waggle it around a little as my lips are dry and I don't want to appear as nervous as I am. A couple brush past on their way into the other quad. I watch them go, arm in arm. Vikki is still staring at me – inscrutable.

I strike another match and bring it to the tip of my cigarette, but as I do so, she blows it out. I'm surprised but her expression doesn't change. She offers no explanation. I take out another match. I light that one, too, but as I bring it to my cigarette, again she blows it out.

Still nothing.

I want to say something but I'm too dazzled. Caught in the moment. I try one last time. I light the match and hold it an inch away from the end of the cigarette, briefly tempting her. She doesn't move a muscle. The match has nearly burned down so I take my eyes off her as I move the match to the tip of the cigarette, satisfied I've called her bluff.

She blows it out once more.

'Coffee?' I say. It's all my addled brain can come up with, and immediately I think it sounds stupid. But she nods.

I turn round and head back into Holywell quad where I live. Half a dozen paces further on I stop to check that she's following. But she's disappeared.

'You want to watch her,' says Robert, one of her fellow historians.

I'm sitting opposite him in the wood-panelled college dining hall at lunchtime. It's long and austere, lined with portraits of former principals, all male and glum-looking. The students walk in, their plates laden from a small outer room where the food is served, and sit randomly at tables arranged on either side.

Robert is a big bluff lad, a northerner. Normally relaxed, on this occasion he seems uncomfortable, shifting around as he speaks, checking that no one is sitting too close. He leans conspiratorially across the table and seems inhibited, almost threatened. 'She's tricky,' he says.

We are joined by a friend of his, Sean, another member of his gang, a group of blokes who all do history and stick together like glue. 'Who are you talking about?' says the newcomer.

'Vikki,' says Robert, cautiously glancing around.

'Oh . . .' The newcomer raises an eyebrow. 'Trouble.' He could be discussing Mata Hari or Madonna. 'Nice but . . . trouble.'

They don't elaborate and I'm left to ponder this strange warning. It makes no sense to me. They are a group of lads who are confident, and not unworldly. Yet somehow they're all wary of this woman.

They don't put me off. Quite the opposite: they pique my interest. Who is this person who troubles them? Intimidates them? Causes them to whisper and lean across the dining-table to warn their fellow man of dire consequences?

I find myself watching her even more closely over the next few days, listening for her name in other people's conversations, noticing its appearances on the college notice-board; sifting the evidence, considering the possibilities, like some obsessive detective who can't stop thinking about a case.

I'm drawn to her, the woman with the exotic eyes and

surname. I watch her come and go around college. I want to know more.

And the more I discover the more intrigued I am. She seems to be an enigma, a contradiction, defying traditional descriptions. She rows well, is in the first eight, though she is neither loud nor hearty; she makes clothes for theatrical productions but is no luvvie; she is not with the popular crowd, the cool kids, the arty Hughs and Alexes, with their Daliesque facial hair and extravagant clothes, their partly written novels, their studied lack of caring. Her best female friend is bright and sporty. Her closest male friends include a brilliant but diffident classicist who expresses his inner turmoil by occasionally thumping people, and a socially awkward but clever languages student from a small Lancashire town who is a self-confessed Coronation Street *addict.*

With her circle of mavericks Vikki, I learn, is part nurturer, part leader, and part agony aunt. At least one of the blokes, if not both, is rumoured to have a crush on her, but she is far too elusive to be pinned down, too busy being herself to be with someone else in a serious way. She tends to deflect any advances – a joke, a comment, a friendly dig and she's away, even as the latest would-be suitor closes in, all serious intent, only to find himself chasing shadows. Or looking for a match to light his cigarette.

Not that she is universally liked: she makes enemies too. There is some eyebrow-raising when I ask someone studying history in another year about her. There is a constant flow of snide comments in the college magazine; she has even, apparently, fallen out spectacularly with her tutor.

Spiky, off centre, unpredictable, fearless, tricky – dangerous, even. An individual who is to be avoided at all costs, according to some. I can't wait for our paths to cross again.

'Cheese and coleslaw jacket potato, please.'

I'm standing some weeks later outside the baked potato van on Oxford High Street. Three vans are huddled together on that stretch of road, providing hot dogs, spuds and burgers. They are neatly parked between a pair of streetlights with three separate queues that snake off into the shadows – the hungry, mostly drunk and desperate strays of a Saturday evening. It is nearly midnight and I am on the way back to my room after playing a gig.

I am in a band, several in fact, and I perform all over town – in colleges, wine bars, the odd pub. I play at birthday parties, summer balls, at eccentric one-off gigs for the Oxford Zoologists, the Geography Society. For a while I have a residency at an Italian restaurant in the centre of town and get paid in pizza.

The music tends to be jazz but all types; standards, jazz rock, some Latin-influenced, some traditional swing. It's always danceable. Crowd-pleasing. Fun. Music with a smile. And it kicks ass.

Without a car, I rely on the other band members to help carry my drums around town. When they aren't available, I use a porter's trolley, a giant flat wooden bed pulled with *a heavy iron bar. I rumble along the pavement, with the drums and cymbals stacked on top (I have no cases), and people have to get out of my way because I can't easily change direction. Every time I slow down at a cross street the drums slide forward and the cymbals clash, like an avant-garde drum solo.*

Drumming has been a passion since I was a boy. It gradually took the place of the historical fancy dress, the 'thinks', so my early adolescence was filled with hours of practice and little else – no girlfriends, no social life, just utter dedication.

I played my first paid gig at fourteen, a Christmas season at a nightclub near Brighton, deputising for my drum teacher, who was working elsewhere and thought it would be good experience for me. The club had low ceilings, dense clouds of cigarette smoke and chicken-in-a-basket dinners. I wore a silk shirt with big puffy sleeves, played two sets a night and occasionally backed the visiting cabaret. There were traditional comedians –

'The money they've made and they still live like pigs.'

'Who's that?'

'Pinky and Perky.'

– country-and-western singers, impressionists and tap-dancing trumpet players.

Other gigs followed my nightclub appearances. I performed at 'Nanny of the Year' at the Wembley Conference centre, and in the orchestra for the musical Cabaret *at a school in Brighton. I even played for the Mid Sussex Symphonia and caused a furore when I screwed up the snare-drum part on 'Land of Hope and Glory'.*

For years, all I wanted to do was play those drums, wherever, whenever. As far as I was concerned my future was mapped out: gigs, recording, fame, sessions, glamour. Joining Genesis as an extra percussionist . . .

Then one day a brilliant new English teacher arrived at my school and introduced me to books. Until then I'd read only drum magazines. Things changed again, at first imperceptibly, then in a headlong rush. My love affair with the drums receded, becoming a fond but distant friendship. I had a new obsession, and before long I was off again on a different path – Shakespeare, Dickens, Thomas Hardy. It was all about words now and the worlds writers could conjure, the fantastic ways that sentences leaped out at you, the images that floated in your mind for hours after you'd met them. A different kind of rhythm.

So I'm not gigging at the Albert Hall right now. I'm not touring with Genesis. I'm not even backing second-rate comedians or tap-dancing trumpet players. I've just played at a student party at Oriel College and am standing in a baked-potato queue on Oxford High Street.

'You want the coleslaw on top of the cheese, yeah?'

'Yes, please.'

'Be a few minutes, the potatoes are like concrete.'

As I wait for my order, I'm thinking about the gig that night, the feeling of playing, the music lifting and surging through the crowd with me at the centre, driving the machine, feeling the energy surge through my arms, my whole body and into my feet, feeling the power, the control, the euphoria, the buzz. The surge is so strong it nails you to the drum stool, the conduit for it all. Immovable. Metronomic.

And I think about the gig that night and the moment it happened. The moment it all started. There is always a particular moment. When you feel the surge start, when it kicks in and you feel your own strength. It's not a particular song, but always a moment in the song when it occurs: the end of a chorus, a key change, the splitting, shrieking high notes at the end of a guitar solo. Then it takes off, slowly at first, like a great weight lifted into the air, slow but easy, as if the great weight was nothing.

I think about the moment that evening, the bridge between Santana's 'Carnaval' and 'Let The Children Play' when the guitar wailed and the drums and percussion started to skip and bounce so irresistibly it was as if I were holding the sticks but they were being manipulated by an invisible player. And I think about looking up through the crude lights and the sweat and the shimmering cymbals, feeling the power go through me and seeing a woman standing at the back of the room, nursing a drink, her head tipped slightly forward so her dark eyes seemed even more hypnotic than ever. The same woman who, a few weeks before, was blowing my matches out.

At that moment, the lights, the colours, the sounds, the

other people receded into the corners of the frame and we were alone in that room, connected by a burst of pure energy, simple and raw, untainted and glamorous. And the moment is frozen. Perfect.

As the moment passed I saw she was standing next to an unusually tall man with a thin, rumpled face and cold, hard eyes. He was trying to talk to her but she seemed more interested in what was happening on stage. At least, I hoped so but I couldn't be sure. Maybe it was just a tactic to avoid talking to him. A few times I knew she was looking at me, and on a couple of occasions I wondered if she was looking at me for a little longer than usual, but when I tried to find her after the gig, she'd disappeared again.

'You were good tonight.'

I turn. She's behind me in the jacket potato queue. 'Thanks,' I reply.

She smiles.

I look around. There's no sign of the tall man. 'Where's . . . ?'

'Him? Just a friend,' she says.

I haven't a clue what to say or do next.

Just then, the queue shuffles up to spare my embarrassment and I am handed my jacket potato.

'Do you want to come and eat that in my room?' she asks.

She lives in a Gothic turret in the older, nineteenth-century, part of the college. There are two interlocking rooms, a small *outer one with a washbasin and, two steps up, a bedroom, with a two-bar electric fire in the corner opposite a single bed. A large barrel of homebrew beer stands on a small table beneath the window. Clothes and papers are strewn about but she seems to know exactly where everything is.*

She hands me a teacup of the beer, which tastes rich and alcoholic, and we sit, me on the edge of the bed, she on the chair next to her desk. We talk and talk . . . Joy Division . . . Leeds United . . . the paintings of Delacroix . . . Jimmy Connors . . . the novels of Graham Greene . . . designing clothes . . . Spencer Tracy . . . the Buzzcocks . . . William Holden . . . Paris.

She is smart, cynical, acerbically funny, and genuine to within an inch of her life.

We talk and laugh, yelp, scream, rock back and forth, agree and disagree, shock each other and clap our hands, 'Yes!' The conversation ebbs and flows and, though, in some ways, we're from opposite ends of the earth – she is the quietly argumentative northerner, with Czech ancestry, whose dad is an engineer while I'm the soft southerner, whose parents met doing am dram – we also have a lot in common; ordinary backgrounds, a state school education and a wariness of the many slick people around us. What's more, we just click.

Within three days I have packed up my few belongings in my rented room and more or less moved into hers. And that's it. We're together. A pair, a team. Through good times and bad, laughter, friendship and adventure, arguments, uncertainty and doubt. Through excitement, discovery and fulfilment, differences, upset and a painful separation. Through the knowledge and realisation that bring you back closer than before. Through the growth pangs of a pair who met when they were barely grown-up. Through the contented years of a couple who know they've made the only sensible choice.

Together: that first summer, in a stifling room in a student house in south Oxford where, on hot summer nights, you have to pour bowls of cold water over yourself to be able to sleep ... In a Masonic Temple where we sleep during the Edinburgh Festival, surrounded by creepy wooden panelling and ceramic eyes that light up ... In a flat in Peckham that is literally sinking – you have to step up a good six inches from the hallway to get to street level ... In the first flat we own in Greenwich, a conversion so small you can put a foot into each room in turn while keeping the other leg anchored in the hall ... In our three-storey cottage just round the corner from that flat where we move most of our possessions with the aid of a wheel-barrow ... In the blue cottage we rent for a summer in Blakeney, Norfolk, with beams so low I hit my head half a dozen times a day ... In the weekend bolt hole we buy in Great Walsingham – an old schoolhouse with a toilet block outside, now converted into a meeting room where, in accordance with the previous owners' wishes, we continue to allow the local Russian Orthodox community to meet for coffee ... In the final home we share, near Holt in

Norfolk, with its quirky garden, muntjac deer, about a million rabbits and a woodland dell stuffed with Day of the Triffids-style plants . . .

Together. Inevitably. Irresistibly. Together.

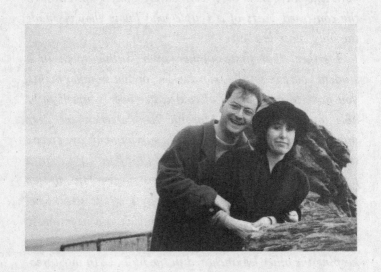

4

A VAST OCEAN

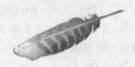

The vicar is a kindly, supportive individual who tries to manage expectations and isn't afraid of sober truth telling. Just occasionally, though, I wish he'd be a little less prosaic.

'It gets worse before it gets better,' he says, of the next few months.

He guides us gently through plans for both services (there is to be a funeral and a memorial) and makes suggestions when we have none. There are hymns to choose as well as readings and poems. Above all there are tributes to write. Lots of words to find. And not just any words but the right words, the perfect words. Words that *capture* her. That *stand* for her. That *represent* her. Words that are *fitting*. That don't let her down. Or *confuse* the reader or listener, that do her *justice*, that strike *the right note*.

Yes, she was sometimes *dogmatic*, but not always, and

wasn't she *belligerent* and *determined* because she *believed in things*? However, if she *believed in things* she wasn't *dogmatic* she was *idealistic* – but, hang on, she could be *dogmatic* as well so I could say that she was *dogmatic sometimes* but *hardly ever*. Maybe I should leave that out if it was *hardly ever* . . . but, then, maybe I should leave it in because otherwise it looks as if I'm trying to put her on a pedestal when she was a *real human being*, with all the flaws that implies. She wasn't just *average* either, or *mundane* – that's not right, far from it. She was a *one-off*. A tremendous person.

I'm drowning in my thoughts and feelings for her. I've put photos everywhere, and cards litter the house. Each morning I go to the post box at the end of my drive and find it jammed with envelopes and packages. They're packed so tightly that the ends of many are crushed when I pull them out. Soon there are so many that the postman abandons the box, comes to the house, knocks on the door and presents me with a thick bundle held together by several elastic bands. From his sombre demeanour, head bowed, wistful, comforting smile, he obviously knows from experience what it all means.

One morning he presents me with a very large pile and I prepare myself for a more than usually tough hour or so. I always open the cards and letters straight away as I feel I must confront them immediately. I cannot let them sit there and fester. That seems like avoidance.

My suspicions were right: this is a particularly difficult day – card after card, letter after letter, all giving voice to the rawest emotions. And I'm wrung out as I read, my chest crushed, my throat dry, my face burning with tears.

As I get to the last envelope, a large brown one, I'm spent, exhausted. I can barely contemplate the huge emotional content that must surely lie within. I sit there for a minute, looking at it, unsure if I can go any further. Then I take a deep breath and pick it up, hand shaking. I tear off the flap and reach inside. My heart is pounding as I lift out the contents. Whatever the emotional conse-quence, I want to get it over quickly now. I have to. I can't take any more of this emotional shellacking. Whatever it says I want to read it and move on but I'm fearful too. I'm scared and on tenterhooks. What more can it say?

I fumble with the contents – it's upside down. Please let it be over. I can't face any more words about how much she meant to you, to me, to all of us. I cannot take any more beautiful personal anecdotes or shared moments or painful reflections on how hard loss is and how difficult my life is almost certainly going to be. I just want to read the thing, put it down and walk out of the room, away from it all. I want to escape. I take one huge breath and focus my eyes on the piece of paper in front of me. I force myself to stare at it, take in those words and absorb them, one last emotional body blow, one last battering among so many. As I cast my eyes down to the text, I wonder what harrowing message it will convey, what heartrending personal testimony it will carry.

It says:

'Think you know Croydon? Think again!'

It's an advertisement for a new housing scheme in south London.

The words from the many cards continue to echo in my head, from the familiar 'With deepest sympathy', 'Words cannot express', 'I was shocked to hear' to the more personal 'Oh my God, Carl' and 'I just cannot believe it'. The cards come in many different shapes: hearts, crosses, some rectangular, some tied with pink string, others edged with borders of flowers, or angels and cherubim. Some are sophisticated and minimalist, others are crudely straightforward. Several are highly individual, one or two are apparently straight off the same shelf at the same high street newsagent. Yet every single one of them is priceless, from the most ornate and sophisticated to the most clichéd and corny. No phrase is wrong, no sentiment misses its mark, no words are inadequate. By their very existence, by the mere fact they were sent, all have huge meaning. They represent a generosity, a kindness on behalf of the sender, a reaching out, an open embracing pair of arms.

There is one message in particular I find myself reciting more often than the rest, over and over again, like a mantra. It seems to say so much about the confusion I feel, the sense of being lost, jolted, thrown, almost unhinged. I return to it time and again. It's a handwritten message shakily scrawled in a card by an elderly friend: 'The older I get, the less I understand.' There's so much confusion still, so much sheer disbelief. Vikki was here but now she is gone. How? How is that possible? Where is she now? Where did she actually go? She can't just have gone. She can't just disappear. She is a person who was alive. How can that not be true? In a moment. In an instant. You can't just *stop*.

The older I get, the less I understand.

The first potential burial site we look at is in the town nearest to where we live. You enter via wrought-iron gates from the main road and then you're into the graveyard straight away, long stretches of lawn dotted with headstones, criss-crossed with gravel paths, the whole place surrounded by a thick hedgerow.

It isn't overlooked but it is on its own, unconnected to a church. It is tidy and neat, but just inside to the left there is a noticeboard that tells you when the gates are shut, that you're not allowed to play loud music and definitely not allowed to picnic there. Or pitch tents. Or bring alcohol. Then you look closer and you see that all the notices are on District Council paper so it's a District

Council burial ground, it will be a District Council burial and a District Council bereavement, and you quickly realise that the only thing you want from your District Council is a decent water supply and someone taking away the bins.

Our local church sits on the top of a rise. Part medieval and part Victorian, it is a survivor of several periods of decay as well as numerous restorations. It looks as if several people, arguing, have built it at the same time, but it's full of character, with its rugged bent roof and old marked stone walls. It isn't ornate and has no pretensions but is, in its own way, mightily impressive.

The graveyard is at the back and looks out over fields on three sides. The fields fall away gradually and you can see for quite some distance across a network of other fields and hedgerows. A tree stands out from the others at the edge of the graveyard. It has died but is still standing, stripped of all its leaves. Its branches, jagged and twisted, reach up dramatically into the huge sky. The graveyard itself is quiet and peaceful; the only sound you can hear is the wind, which whistles at you across the landscape.

This is the place.

The day of the funeral has a dreamlike quality, as if it never happens. I remember only moments, snapshots: the shocking sight of the coffin just sitting at the front of the church when I arrive; my daughter, Romy, shivering in the cold wind as I cradle her next to the grave; the crude thump of the earth as it lands on the coffin courtesy of the gravediggers as they fill in the hole. Couldn't they have been a bit gentler?

Then we walk away as the crisp, clear air whips across the fields and up the hill, and the vicar tells me, pointing across at the soil now piled up high, 'She's not there, you know.'

And although I know what he means, I'm also angry. Angry because it feels as if he's somehow diminishing the ceremony. Have we all been playing out a charade?

Whilst we've been at the church the school PTA, of which Vikki was the head, have adorned the dining room back at the house with flowers and food. There are plates of quiche, pies, sandwiches, salads, and displays of roses and lilies, a stunning sight to greet us on our return.

In twos and threes the mourners arrive and mill around awkwardly in the hallway. Fearful of saying the wrong thing, they talk in hushed tones, leaning in to each other, whispering, like conspirators. Apart from the children, that is. Soon they're rushing around as normal, playing games, clattering up the staircase, thundering around on the landing.

Slowly the day unwinds. As more alcohol is consumed, people relax and the conversations become louder. Emotions, largely reined in at the beginning, now start to pour out. People hug. I go to offer a middle-aged mourner a drink and find he's suddenly crying in the arms of his wife. Elsewhere, someone laughs uproariously at a joke about a badly behaved relative at a funeral.

As evening draws nearer, the weather closes in. The wind that was cold earlier and cut across the graveside now rolls itself up into a howling gale. Biblical grey clouds fill the sky. Then it all stops and the sky clears as it gets dark. Most spectacularly, a single shooting star appears.

A friend points it out. 'That's her,' he says.

For my part I'm just manically busy, absorbed in various routines, marshalling everyone, organising taxis to the station, getting orders for the takeaway Indian meal in the evening, ensuring everyone has a full glass, doing introductions, making small talk.

I find myself trying to make the day go well, which seems very important to me. I'm honouring someone who made all kinds of events go really well and I want to do the same. I don't want to let her down.

I want to throw a good funeral.

I stay alert and attend to the needs of my guests. I don't drink too much, and when it's over, I have a curious sense of a job reasonably well done. Of course I know that the more I think about topping up glasses and handing out napkins, the more I worry about how people are getting home and who ordered the onion bhaji, then the more I can avoid the sheer awfulness of it all, the fact that I'm welcoming people into my house because my wife has died at the age of forty-four, leaving me and our daughter alone, her parents devastated, her sister bereft, her friends shocked and all of us wondering where on earth is the justice in any of it.

So, I stick with the glasses and the taxis and the take-away menus, and don't engage with the reality of it. I don't go near it. Who could? It's too vast to contemplate. An ocean stretching out to the horizon.

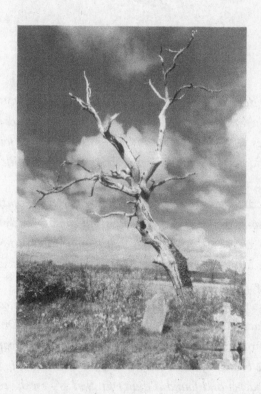

5

HIGHER AND HIGHER

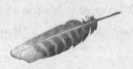

An incident makes Vikki laugh, and I think it says a lot about her. And me. And our relationship. It reduces her to hysterics when it happens and remains a constant source of mirth down the years, guaranteed to make her smile every time it's mentioned.

It occurs on a day when I haven't been concentrating, which some would say is most days, but I'm a comedy writer and the characters and stories that float around in my head tend to limit my grasp of everyday reality, at least during working hours.

Earlier, I have picked up my suit from the dry cleaners and placed it on the bed in its polythene cover. On a tea break from script writing, I have absentmindedly wandered into the bedroom, taken out the suit from its wrapping, tried on the jacket and found it didn't fit. So I try on the trousers and they too feel unfamiliar.

There is no other explanation as far as I'm concerned. It's the wrong suit.

I'm so caught up in the moment, so obsessed with the sheer injustice of it all, that I have one thought: to have it out with the dry cleaners who have given me someone else's clothes.

I tear down the road, still wearing the jacket and trousers. 'This suit isn't mine,' I say, as I barge in.

'Which suit?' the woman behind the counter replies.

'The one I'm wearing,' I say.

She looks at me, a little confused. 'So the suit you're wearing isn't yours?'

'No,' I continue. 'It doesn't fit.'

There is a pause.

'The suit you're missing. What label is it?' she asks.

I look inside the one I'm wearing. It says 'Woodhouse'.

'This one,' I say, recognising the name.

'And what colour is your suit, sir?'

I look down at it. Now she mentions it, the colour looks familiar too.

'This colour,' I reply. Something is definitely dawning on me.

She looks me up and down. 'Is it possible Sir might just have put on a bit of weight?' I notice the corners of her mouth curl up into the start of a smile.

I look at my jacket and trousers, then at the woman behind the counter and I realise that this is, without doubt, my suit. I start to make for the door and the only thing I can think of to say at this juncture, the only face-saving, dignity-preserving aside I can come up with, is: 'I think I need to speak to my wife.'

Then I walk out of the door.

There are several reasons why Vikki finds this story funny. She likes it because it's a little off-beat and quirky and that appeals to her sense of humour. It is not the story of someone being witty or droll or superior or smart – that's not the kind of thing that makes her laugh. It's the story of someone being human and frail and bonkers.

It's also apparently quite 'me' and she likes the parts of me it reveals: the capacity to be totally convinced of something, oblivious as to whether it makes me look like an idiot; my tendency to sail away on a tide of what many might regard as near insanity; a complete inability, even when I've realised I'm in the wrong, to climb down in anything approaching a polished manner. And then there is my rare talent, right at the end of a crisis, for signing off with the most toe-curling farewell imaginable, of which 'I think I need to speak to my wife' is only an average example.

To sum up, she likes this story because it shows I'm rubbish. And she likes the fact that I'm rubbish. And most of all she likes the fact that I haven't a clue how to hide it.

She believes in the honesty of that. Of being yourself, horrible, mind-numbing social catastrophes and all. She hates the falseness of people pretending, covering, disguising. Wherever she goes, whatever she does, Vikki is proudly, irreducibly, vulnerably herself. It is one of the things she looks for in other people, and finds in me; the man with someone else's suit.

The incident at the dry cleaners took place in Greenwich, which is not where our London lives began . . .

Post-university our first destination is Peckham, the joyless concrete and dreary Peckham of the mid-eighties, not the gentrified London village of today. At the time we don't notice its rough edges – we're still living as we did at college: late nights, parties, turning up for work with red eyes and a sore head. Crucially we retain the self-absorbed naivety that most students possess: we just accept the angry atmosphere in the town centre, the tensions on the night bus. When there is a fight in the local kebab shop while we're ordering food, we're initially shocked but joking about it by the time we get home.

Vikki is working at a bank. It's mundane and low level, not what she wants to do, but at least it's regular work, something to tide her over during this uncertain, post-college phase when she's still trying to work out where she's heading. I'm sending off stacks of material to Private Eye, *then watching it come back a week or so later with a note, saying, 'We recommend you send this to* Punch.'

I'm also working up a live comedy act with a partner and testing it out on the fledgling alternative cabaret circuit. I perform at a variety venues across London; a club just outside the Blackwall Tunnel, a small theatre in Maida Vale, the back room of a pub on a Sunday lunchtime where they pass a jug round and people put in coins. We perform on bills of three or four acts, all competing to be the headliner or the one just after the interval when everyone has had a bit to drink and is properly warmed up. The acts themselves are varied: a wild assortment of single comics, duos, jugglers, satirical singers, poets, ventriloquists, impressionists, a Marxist magic act and a man who puts fireworks up his bottom and lights them.

Vikki is invariably there after work or at weekends and always sits at the back of the audience. When I get on stage, I look for her through the lights and the fug of smoke. There she is, alone, nursing a drink. Self-contained. In her own world. Just as she was at that very first gig.

Despite the unprepossessing surroundings, she never questions my enthusiasm. She never asks where it's all going, though in those early days she has every right to doubt. She never wonders why she is invariably the one paying the rent at home, she just sits there, quietly supporting me. If it goes well, we celebrate. If it's been a disaster, she's wonderfully adept at tending my wounds.

The place we rent, along with a couple of friends in Peckham, is a typical first flat, on the ground floor of a badly converted Victorian house. It consists of a narrow corridor off which there are three bedrooms. There is also a small bathroom and a living room, which contains a primitive kitchen. The whole place is dark and smells musty because the only windows of any size in the whole place look out onto a small enclosed concrete backyard. The man who owns the house is a Greek builder and uses the yard to store various bits of equipment. Should you wish to fling open the curtains to let in some light, it is not unusual to find yourself confronted by the sight of forty toilet seats.

With these surroundings it is not surprising that we go out as much as possible, even though we don't have much money, and when we discover the Montague Arms, a big cheap pub on a noisy section of the nearby Old Kent Road, we quickly make that our centre of operations. It becomes the focus of many mid-eighties evenings, a place where we meet friends or spend whole evenings by ourselves, away from the airless bunker that is just around the corner. It's a home from home, a place where we drink cheap lager, eat egg and chips, and debate Thatcher's foreign policy or whether mobile phones will ever catch on.

The Montague Arms is a pub with a difference. It doesn't have one theme but many, possibly all the themes that have ever been dreamed of. Its walls are festooned with skeletons, coffins, scarecrows, assorted weapons and a rowing boat. There are animal horns, bits of armour and shop signs hanging from the ceiling so you have to continually duck your head. To one side of the bar you can see the front end of a Mini that looks as if it has just crashed through the wall. The overall effect is part dazzling, part weird, as if the pub has just been bought by a prop designer who has taken too much LSD.

There is a stage at one end of the room and a duo from

Yorkshire play top-twenty hits dwarfed by an array of instruments that would be the envy of any stadium-filling prog-rock group. The keyboard player is blind and the drummer is an egomaniac who throws in completely unsuitable drum fill-ins on simple numbers – imagine Buddy Rich playing 'Happy Birthday'.

Occasionally, when the keyboard player, Les, doesn't feel the audience (normally a coachload of Dutch tourists) is sufficiently enthusiastic, he offers encouragement, which takes the form of aggressively shouting, 'Come on, you buggers!'

The Montague seems to typify those early years in Peckham. It started out as a really novel and fun place and we often took people there, saying things like 'You won't believe this bar we've found!' But then, after a while, it became routine and tiresome as we bobbed and wove our way around the room trying to avoid the decorations and being yelled at by Les. It had a garish excitement about it, an immediate novelty value, but it was only skin deep. At the end of the day it was just two middle-aged blokes from Yorkshire playing top twenty hits rather poorly in a tourist bar and we were starting to want something more substantial.

For we were changing, shaking off our student chains. It was that time, mid- to late-twenties. We started to want a modicum of comfort, privacy, a space of our own, something more than a builder's yard at the back and the owner barging in on a Saturday morning demanding his rent.

∗   ∗   ∗

One by one the other people in the flat leave to buy their first homes and we are left with increasingly empty, increasingly dilapidated surroundings. We don't belong there any more. We begin to feel that life is going on elsewhere – more exciting, more rewarding, just better.

Sometimes when we're feeling flush we get a minicab up the road to Greenwich and have a curry in a cosy Indian restaurant with booths, picturing a time when we can live there – we both have an affinity with the place, having been visited on day trips as kids.

We like its village feel, its market, its history, its beautiful park – that it doesn't have the snobby air of other similar parts of London. Greenwich is classy, different and yet down to earth. It's eccentric and individual and has its own glamour but it doesn't shout too loud. We hope it's a bit like us. I know it's a lot like Vikki.

Over our Friday night curries we dream and plot, and she brings out her gigantic eighties calculator the size of a cricket scoreboard, and with her usual wizardry and enthusiasm works it all out. No unnecessary shopping, home-cooked food and nights in watching Hill Street Blues. *Then we can just about afford to buy.*

After eighteen months of scrimping, saving and borrowing, we finally make the move, a new conversion opposite the station, a tiny flat where the bedroom is so small there's barely space for the bed – we have to fold it up and store it during the day. But we're excessively proud of the place and we fuss over it, and she gets in Ikea shelves and persuades a man at John Lewis to give us an ex-display wardrobe for a fraction of the real price, and we're proper home owners.

What's more, the move invigorates us. It's as if our new surroundings have conferred on us a new stature. I start to taste a little success, writing and performing on the radio, getting some sitcoms on TV. Vikki too starts to really make her mark working for a high-street retailer. Suddenly, from drifting in and out of various jobs, it's as if she's really found herself and things start to fall into place. She is focused, bustling with brilliant energy. She has always been interested in clothes – hence the costume designing at Oxford – and now she has found a way to follow her passion. The environment suits her too. It is fast-paced, demanding and uses her skill; an ability to organise people, inspire them, and make them work more efficiently. She is good with numbers as well.

Over the next few years she rises inexorably through the ranks, always in her quiet, unassuming way, without fanfare or fuss. There are no celebratory parties or overly excitable phone calls when she gets a promotion. On occasion I have to drag it out of her. From very junior buyer to merchandiser to senior merchandiser then director of merchandising in the blink of an eye. She starts to travel too – Hong Kong, China, Paris.

She gets picked out for a special EU project – the British representative on an international panel, travelling all over Europe looking at the future of retail – Berlin, Lausanne,

Helsinki, Amsterdam, Denmark. Still no fuss. No fanfare. Just being herself. Being good at it all.

She becomes a senior executive and still manages to do it her way. Doesn't change just because she's moved up in the world. She is friendly with those who bring the tea into meetings. She has no airs or haughtiness. No front. No bullshit. She doesn't feel the need to put on an act. She's just herself – honest and cynical with a dislike of superiority and those of a flashy disposition: the blokey executives who bang the table and act macho; the cocky suppliers with their champagne nights out, and their Hertfordshire swagger. That makes her cross, and when she gets cross she goes very Yorkshire and mutters under her breath: 'Fookin' tosser.' Like a grizzled miner or hard-bitten club cricketer on a cold day at Scarborough. 'Fookin' tosser.'

It's 1997. Vikki's career has gone through the roof with a new senior post at a national retail outlet. She is at the peak of her profession. She is a whirlwind of energy, ideas and resourcefulness. She's happy. And we are happy too – excited by life, by the climb through our thirties into prosperity, with adventure and fun on the way. Lots of socialising, impulsive trips abroad, that delicious unencumbered time, when possibilities stretch endlessly ahead, like beacons, and life is anything we want it to be.

Her success is rubbing off on me too: after years of knocking on the door, working on shows for other people, my own series on BBC2 is commissioned. Suddenly the gigs in scruffy pubs seem a long time ago as Stressed Eric, *the first adult British animated sitcom about the most stressed individual in the world, takes wing, and we're both soon dashing for planes that take us in opposite directions halfway round the world.*

She is in Hong Kong, buying for her company. I am in Los Angeles working on my show with Klasky Csupo, makers of The Simpsons, *and we meet for passion-filled weekends at the Royalton in New York and never leave the hotel room. Our lives are suddenly a living, breathing Sunday supplement, full of glamour and colour, madness and adventure. It's as if Fortune has smiled on us and we are blessed and lucky, and some divine being has reached out his hand and beckoned us closer, and we are moving onwards and upwards, higher and higher.*

It is a February evening when I land back in the UK. Production has wrapped on the series and I've been meeting American networks who might be interested in broadcasting the show. Vikki has collected me at the airport and we've headed straight to our favourite Italian restaurant in Blackheath. It's balmy and the skies are clear as we park the car and head inside. Vikki has been quiet on the return journey and I've been doing all the talking; I'm wired and exhausted, jubilant and a little confused.

It normally takes a few days for me to reconnect and it isn't just the jetlag, more the sense of trying to slot back into a different life. Over there it's all just about the show and

I'm totally selfish. When I get back I have to be a husband again, to think of someone else once more. Vikki calls it reprogramming me.

Now I'm out of whack, certainly, maybe more so than usual. All I can think of is what I have left behind – Ari Emmanuel, the inspiration for the fictional Ari Gold in Entourage *and one of the biggest agents in the US, is representing me to the networks in the States and I am in a state of tingling excitement. What's more, I've just found out we have offers for the show from two of the majors. Vikki still seems subdued as I continue to chatter away and, as we settle at our favourite table near the window, it feels as if we're an ocean apart.*

'There's something I need to talk about,' she suddenly says.

'Do you realise what this means? Competing offers!'

I'm still breathless with my own excitement.

'— Can I just say something?' she says.

I interrupt her: 'It is a bidding war!'

'Look, Carl—'

'I know but just let me finish. It is a bidding war, okay? Do you know how rare that is?'

I'm still mentally ten thousand miles away. She looks harassed. I'm cross with her. She doesn't seem to be hearing what I have to say. When the wine comes, she pours it a little too rapidly and won't let go of the bottle. Still I'm away in a world of my own.

'With Fox I'd be on the same network as The Simpsons *which would be fabulous but NBC are the biggest broad-*

caster in the world. What a great choice to have. Don't you think?'

Suddenly she leans forward and says, in a loud voice, 'I'm trying to talk to you!'

Several heads turn in the restaurant. This isn't like Vikki at all. She's normally a quiet, restrained individual. She can be cross and bossy but would never normally cause a scene. Then I look at her hand and notice it's gripping the bottom of the wine bottle hard. And shaking.

'There is a lump,' she says. 'I've found a lump.'

6

THE MAN WHO COULDN'T GET OVER IT

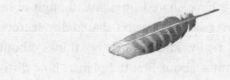

There's a man who couldn't get over the fact that I'm a widower. He sees me as soon as I rush into the chemists some days after the funeral. He is queuing for the cashier, who is right by the door when I enter the shop. I can't slip in unnoticed. I can't creep past him. I can't pretend I haven't noticed he's there. I have to stop and talk. I'm aware it might be awkward for him. I'm not the person I was when I last saw him for he didn't come to the funeral, and I haven't seen him at all since my wife's death. My status has now changed: I was a married man but now I'm a widower. And we both have to deal with that.

The man who couldn't get over it is not someone I know well but we're more than acquainted. He is a school parent, like me, and I have picked up my daughter when he has picked up his, waited alongside him in the foyer of draughty dance studios next to him, stood gossiping next to him on netball touchlines. We've spoken about art, writing, cars, football, though none of it in depth. We've got beneath the surface – a little. We know what we think about certain things but only certain things. We have shared opinions, though none have been controversial. We haven't shared any secrets, though. I don't really know what he thinks about anything important – about life, the planet, how difficult it is to be a father. And he's certainly not a close friend – even allowing for the woolly, insubstantial nature of most male friendships. I would say he's someone I know a bit, a bloke I'm friendly with, though not a friend. Someone I'm matey with, although I wouldn't go so far as to say he was a mate either. I'd call him if I had a problem with my car. I certainly wouldn't call him if I had a problem with my soul.

Still, there's something there. Something at stake. Something that means this encounter matters.

By the look on his face you can tell that my sudden appearance is a shock. He wasn't expecting this – maybe a conversation with the old lady behind him about the state of the weather or a casual exchange with the young mum in front about the problems of parking in Holt.

But no.

He is face to face with the Widower.

And I know he knows that immediately because I can

see that look in his eyes, a look of terror and embarrassment.

Maybe if he'd had some warning about my appearing in the shop it would have been okay. He could have prepared something to say. Practised it. Tested it out on his wife, or one of his friends. Better still, they could have just *told* him what to say since, like most blokes, I suspect that bereavement really isn't his thing. But he's been caught horribly unaware.

And he's face to face with the Widower.

The man who couldn't get over it goes red immediately. A deep crimson red. Red that glows and throbs in his cheeks as if someone is controlling them with bellows. He shrugs. He touches my arm. He tuts. He looks at the floor, then back at me. He opens his mouth. Nothing comes out. 'If I . . .' he begins.

I look hopeful.

He tries again. 'If I . . . if I can . . .'

'Yes?' I reply.

But nothing comes out.

'If I . . .'

He was closer the first time.

'Really, if I . . .' he continues.

There is a pause. He's straining every sinew but can't speak. I try to help him out. 'I know,' I say.

But he's determined to go on. 'I'm so . . .' He looks fit to explode.

'Absolutely,' I add.

'I'm totally . . .' He opens his mouth wider, absurdly wide, as if there is a greater chance of some words slipping out if the hole is bigger.

I lean forward, willing him on.

'You know I . . .'

'I completely understand,' I say.

He takes a deep breath. 'So as I was saying . . .'

'No, really. I completely understand.'

'You know I . . .'

'I do. Really I do.'

A beat.

He just stands there looking at the floor.

Is it over? Hopefully. Maybe. Is the torture at an end?

Of course it isn't. Because he's a bloke and he isn't a quitter and won't give up, and it's probably the same as when he said he'd put up that Ikea wardrobe in twenty minutes because it was so bloody easy, then found he was struggling with it two days on but refused to get someone else to take over. No, he's darned well going to say his piece.

So on it goes. He starts to speak again, then clams up. I nod encouragingly at him and try to draw him out, which doesn't work. Time passes. Deodorants and hair ties are purchased behind us. Still he remains.

If someone hadn't opened the door of the shop at some point and called his name, I think he'd still be there, years on, locked in his own hellish Groundhog Day, caught in a web of embarrassment and shyness, unable to communicate in any way because he fears communicating in the wrong way.

Instead, he stumbles out of the shop, making the sign of a telephone back at me, and runs when he gets through the door. I am left alone with my thoughts, looking at the cashier, who stares back at me in utter confusion.

I still see the man who couldn't get over it. We pass each other in the high street from time to time or end up queuing behind each other in shops in the town – it's not the kind of place where you can disappear. And I can honestly say that he's still never got over the shock of seeing me in that shop because whenever I meet him now exactly the same thing happens: his face goes ruby red and he is suddenly reduced to that strange, stuttering, catatonic state.

No matter what I say or how differently I start the conversation – 'Norwich doing well, aren't they?' hardly sounds to me like an invitation to talk about death – he seems compelled to return to the conversation he couldn't complete in the first place, to go back just once more in case, with the passage of time, by some miracle, he finds he can break through, conquer his stumbling uncertainties and finally spit it out.

But he can't, and his latest attempt is just added to the litany of failure. Another piece of baggage weighing him down, the next time he attempts it. As he surely will. He can't help it. It's the force of history, the way he's been programmed.

And as he sprints hurriedly away from me or crosses the road to avoid me or suddenly accelerates past me when he sees me coming towards him as he now tends to do (and, to be honest, I do as well), I always think back to that first encounter and the bizarre ways that bereavement changes relationships forever.

7

TELLING

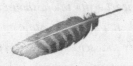

You always know there's something wrong because they call the partner in, if they're waiting outside.

They call the partner in, and you go into the room and it's quiet, even though a number of people are there – various nurses, the consultant. But they're quiet for a reason. They're quiet because they're just waiting. Waiting till everyone's present before they say it.

I see Vikki's frightened face. That's all I can see as I walk in. She's sitting at the end of the hospital bed in her gown. She looks hunched and frail. Her voice has an awful strangled quality to it. 'Carl. What is it? Carl?'

I go over to her and sit next to her. My throat is so tight I can't speak but I take her hand. It feels cold and her whole body is shivering.

'Oh, no,' she says. 'No.'

Someone has closed the door behind me and the nurses

and the consultant now form a rough semi-circle round the bed. They are all staring at us, poised, ready to react, ready to move in, ready to catch us if we fall.

'Oh, God,' says Vikki.

And time seems to slow down as the consultant speaks, and instantly I feel my heart erupt into a thousand rapid beats and a tidal wave of adrenaline crashes into me, a furious, angry rush within my body that scrambles my nerves but overwhelms my capacity for conscious thought in a body that is already shutting down. I am paralysed and alive at the same time, strong and feeble, barely conscious and horribly awake.

I look at her and she looks so helpless, her lips cracked, dry and open. All colour has gone from her face and her arms. I feel us being pulled apart. Separated. Even while we are still holding hands.

Afterwards we take a long, circuitous walk home past familiar places, places we've passed a hundred times. But now they seem different, shrouded in a fog, their colours dimmed, their sounds muffled. And we can barely feel our own footsteps as we trudge home. Past the Trafalgar pub on the Thames, with its beautiful upstairs room where we held our wedding reception, the sun shining through the old windows at the guests, nearly all in their twenties too, setting out on life, bright, optimistic and fearless. Along the river walk, with the Queen's House in the background and the hill at the top of the park climbing behind it into the sky, where we sat, picnicked and drank in the world. Past the Cutty Sark *where we held a home-made engagement party, carrying our bottles of wine and glasses onto the boat in cardboard boxes. Past the Fan museum, past the house of Cecil Day-Lewis, past the old theatre, past our favourite restaurant, with its crisp white tablecloths, its black bread, herring and vodka starter, and pictures of old vaudevillians, its sense of old London. Past the gates of Greenwich park where we shared an ice cream on one of our very first visits – having taken the riverboat on an impossibly glorious summer's day from Embankment, two excited, impoverished students from Peckham putting the world to rights. Through our favourite spot, the formal gardens near the iron gates onto Crooms Hill and 'our' seat top right in the corner. Down King George Street, scene of a thousand Sunday strolls. Home to our house round the corner, which we'd left two hours earlier – different people, looking forward to different lives.*

Our Greenwich. Our home. Where we grew up together. Where we became us. Where Vikki was told she had breast cancer.

'Are you going to start or shall I?' I ask.

'I will, then you can step in if it gets difficult,' she says.

The train is rumbling north to Leeds. The two of us are sitting, with her sister Patricia, in a packed carriage, trying not to be too loud. It's a Saturday in May, though there is a distinct chill in the air.

'I'll start with the fact that I've had an operation. And that's done,' continues Vikki.

'That's good, so the problem is in the past,' adds Patricia, trying to sound encouraging.

'Absolutely,' says Vikki. 'And then I'll say about the chemo coming up.'

'You sure you don't want me to say anything, just to help out?' I ask.

'Oh, God, I don't know. Maybe. I don't know. Just let me start. Then . . .'

'Then if you can't speak any more, I'll come in,' I add.

'Yes. Okay. Let's see . . . maybe . . .'

Vikki is full of doubts. I can see her confidence just draining away. I want the moment to come quickly now. Come quickly and be over.

'Not too much detail,' I say.

'No,' she says. 'We need to emphasise that the prospects of a full recovery are good. We've had the operation to remove the lump, and they've taken out some lymph nodes, and only a tiny number are affected, which is good.'

'Which is very good,' says Patricia.

'Very good,' I repeat decisively, positively.

Vikki nods.

'It'll be fine,' I say, as firmly and as confidently as I can.

'Absolutely,' adds Patricia.

I lean across to take Vikki's hand. It is cold and fragile.

We are telling people. We are breaking into their lives and changing them forever.

'Hi, I didn't expect to see you?'

'No, it's just there's something I've got to tell you – I've got cancer.'

Breaking into their lives and changing them forever.

Vikki wants to tell both sets of parents in one weekend. She wants to make it quick and tell them one after the other. Leeds, then Sussex. Face to face. In and out. Tell them, leave them and give them a chance to regroup, to contemplate, to help each other. We have to do it, we have to. It feels like the bit at the end of The Godfather, we joke grimly on the train as we near our destination. Quick. Swift. Brutal. Bang-bang. One murderous visitation after another.

This is the way Vikki wants to play it. This is the only way because it is her way. No fuss, no hoo-hah, no distractions. She has had to concentrate on the cancer, on her operation, on her survival, on herself. Others have had to wait. Until now.

The train rattles a little as it turns and threads its way past the familiar tall tower blocks on the outskirts of Leeds. Slowly it curves as it eases into the centre and I feel my chest tighten as it bends into the heart of the city.

A few weeks before we are in the basement of the hospital in the anaesthetic room.

Vikki is lying on a hospital trolley waiting to be put to sleep. This is part one of the treatment, the operation, the lumpectomy, when the cancer cells will be removed, when the *evil will be extracted. She just wants it out. We both want it gone as fast as possible. At this stage only Patricia and I and a couple of friends know.*

I am staying with Vikki in her room upstairs in the hospital and have come down with her in the lift, holding her hand as the porter pushed her. We haven't spoken for the last half an hour as we're both too nervous. We've just held hands.

We hold hands a lot now. We have done almost continuously since the diagnosis. We sit for hours at home just holding hands when inspiration has dried up, when quiet is preferable to anything else. We hold hands when we go to hospital for consultations. We hold hands while she is being examined, even if I have to stick my arm through a curtain. At night at home we just lie on the bed, hold hands and stare at the ceiling. It says so much.

We're together still. We won't be parted. I'm here. I won't let you go. I'll help. I'll give you strength. I'll help you beat this. Together we'll do it. Don't forget, together we'll beat this.

I never realised before, the power of holding hands. It's worth a thousand words. Now as she lies on the trolley, it's worth a million.

'How long does it take before I'm out?' she asks the anaesthetist.

'I think the record is five seconds,' he replies, in a jovial manner.

I chuckle nervously and squeeze her hand. I know from

the way her eyes flash across at me that she's frightened but she's hiding it well.

'I can beat that record any day,' she says, with a smile.

'Excellent,' he says. 'I'm going to count down now.'

He stares intently at her as he feeds the anaesthetic in. 'Five, four, three . . .' He stops, and as I look down at her, I see she has drifted off already. 'Oh, well, better luck next time,' he says, smiling.

He looks at me. 'Okay, then . . . Mr Gorham?'

It's time for me to go and I back out of the door of the anaesthetic room. Just before I leave, I see them open the double doors on the opposite side and deliver her into the operating theatre. I feel as if I've lost her.

As I walk out of the door and into the corridor, I start to cry.

The train is now well into Leeds, passing Elland Road, the football ground where we've been many times. I look at the vast cantilevered stand that cuts into the sky and think of how that immense sturdy sight always excites me, fills me with the warmth of anticipation. It always did until now. Now it's just a sickening reminder of something else. The fact that we're approaching the moment. The next time we pass the stadium, on the way out, her parents will know.

The taxi ride from the station to where they live is completed in total silence. As we get out, it feels eerie: the house is a picture of neatness, with its clipped front garden and immaculate row of flowers.

As we arrive we go straight into the living room and sit down because we have our news to impart. Then there is an awful moment when Vikki tries to usher her parents into the room so they're there at the same time. They obviously haven't a clue what is to come so they're flitting in and out, the way that people do when you first arrive – bringing tea and remembering cake, nipping back to collect napkins.

Worse still, in their innocence, they're smiling and joking, even at one point deliberately leaving the room in mock rebellion as Vikki's request to sit down becomes more and more insistent.

It's a shocking, cruel scenario.

I don't recall exactly what is said when they finally settle . . .

It happens, is all I know. In a blur, in a cloud. Our scripted, rehearsed version falls apart quite quickly, and Vikki dries early on so I find myself stepping in. Maybe because they're not my parents it's easier for me to talk, to master the dryness in my throat, my shaking hands and my tight chest. But I'm slightly surprised at how calm and measured I appear to sound.

I mention the operation she's just had, the chemo to come, the positive outlook. I don't go into much detail for there is no need: it's big enough as it is.

Vikki's mother, a tiny, redoubtable woman, sits and listens intently, stoically. Her gaze doesn't waver. She doesn't flinch.

She just takes it all in . . . As if someone told her what to expect seconds before and she had just enough time to marshal her defences.

Vikki's father, on the other hand, a big, tall Lancastrian, looks immediately crushed. His eyes show terrible surprise, then vulnerability. And after, just desolation.

At the end there is a silence and I sense their world spinning away from their grasp, out of reach now, somewhere on the horizon. It will take them a long time to catch it up, to get it back and secure it once more, if they ever can.

Vikki, Patricia and I feel helpless. For now we must let them drift to find their own salvation. Now we have told them, we can't do any more; we can't take away their pain; we can't stop them feeling devastated; we just have to leave them to contemplate it.

Part of me almost feels guilty at what we've done – our shocking act of vandalism – the way we've busted in on a clear summer's afternoon to this innocent corner of Yorkshire and wrecked their lives with this bombshell right out of the blue. But it's the best we can do. It's the best anyone could do.

Cancer is like that. You take the best option you can and it's still pretty shitty.

After a while and several silent, shocked embraces, we get up and leave. There's no doubt that this is the right time for us to go. No one feels inclined to go back to small talk. So we leave them, glassy-eyed, like statues at the end of their drive, staring after us, the terrible executioners, off on another mission.

* * *

'*Are you okay?*'

'*I'm okay.*'

'*What about you?*'

We smile at each other but there's nothing much left behind the smiles.

Next day, Vikki and I are getting out of the car outside the flats in Sussex where my parents live. We're going to do this one by ourselves, just the two of us. It is a beautiful morning. I can feel the sun's heat on my face as I shut the car door. It seems so strange. The flowers are starting to bloom. The bushes near the front door are a rich green and full of life. Everything is shiny and warm and optimistic. This isn't the kind of thing you should be doing on a day like this.

This is part two, though, and we can't escape it. The second time we have to deliver the poisonous news. The second time to feel sick and full of dread as we approach a familiar door.

We've amended our script, tweaked and honed it on the way down. Like a pair of actors, we've tried to learn from the audience response first time round. Tried to make it better. We've convinced ourselves we're veterans now. That we know what works. We've told ourselves we should feel more confident this time. It can't feel as bad as it did the first time. Surely.

But it does. And in some ways it's worse because we've already been through this once, and seeing the shocked faces, the lost expressions, the sheer desolation yet again is a horrible reminder and eats away at our already depleted, near-exhausted reserves of emotion.

This time there is no farcical preamble. Both of my parents are there, in the living room. Both are sitting quietly, ready for something, though they have no idea what. And soon we're in the midst of it again, the awful shocking revelation that tears at them and us as sharply as a jagged nail on the arm.

This time it is me who breaks down. No sooner have I started, than my throat closes up and all I can give out are great huge thumping sobs. I try several times to start again but I have to admit defeat. Vikki takes back the reins and somehow we get through it.

My parents' reaction mirrors that of the others almost exactly. My mother absorbs the shock without flinching. Within seconds she is asking practical questions about her role as a supporter, while my father looks fragile, like a lost boy, almost swept away by the news. It's as if the women seem somehow programmed to cope, as if there is an unconscious, intuitive resource that kicks in at the mention of the words 'breast cancer'. In contrast the men seem completely overwhelmed, confused, bereft.

It is Vikki who outlines the process this time. She talks about the operation that has been and gone, the chemotherapy, the positive outlook. All the time my mum nods gently, hands folded whilst my father just stares, eyes wide. Vikki does a great job of being the calmer one this time, the one who masters the shaking hands and overcomes the hoarseness in her voice.

As before, when the speaking stops we get up and go quite quickly. We leave them to their own consolations and doubtless long, agonised phone calls with the other set of parents.

The sun has gone in, replaced by clouds, as we walk down the steps outside their flat. It's raining gently and there's a distinct breeze. It's good to feel the breeze. We've been hot and sweaty with tension for so much of the last forty-eight hours.

As we drive away we reflect on the tortuous, bizarre and difficult weekend we've just had. It has tested us to the limit, strained every sinew, shaken every single emotion till it has begged for mercy. It has challenged us, terrified us, made us search deep inside ourselves. It has made us contemplate our lives and somehow brought us closer. Both of us feel exhausted, but curiously proud. Both of us are aware that this is only the start.

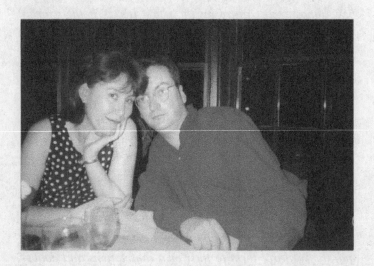

8

THE BUSINESS OF GRIEF

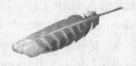

The food has stopped. That's how you know time has passed. The food has stopped appearing on my doorstep. It started a few weeks after the funeral – shepherd's pie, boeuf bourguignon, various casseroles, all neatly wrapped in foil containers, with instructions written in pencil on the lid. They appeared without fanfare, without any kind of announcement, from a couple of kind neighbours – a practical and thoughtful gesture, though one that made me reflect on the oddness of my new situation. In the strange, inverted sexist world of the bereaved, it seems men are not expected to be able to fend for themselves in even the most basic ways.

But it's three months on and the food has stopped. Also, people in general have ceased asking me how I am. Now if they meet me, they just smile a little wanly, then change the subject or go, 'Tsk,' as if to say, 'Oh dear, we're still sorry but we're finding it a bit difficult to know what to say now. Can we possibly talk about something else?' Put simply, other people have moved on with their lives and I haven't.

And I can well understand them. In the normal world, things happen and then they pass. There is progress, change and everyone moves forward. But bereavement isn't like that. It lurks. It stays. It hangs around. It's one big drag. A gigantic bore. Immovable, relentless, unyielding. Always there. Every day. Same bloody thing.

You can't *do* anything with bereavement. You can't make it go away or speed it up or pretend it's something else or disguise it as something better. It's just there – weighty and tedious. It doesn't really change from day to day or week to week. It takes months or years to alter in any meaningful way.

And after a while this is a problem for the non-bereaved. A big problem. Hard to understand. Hard to deal with. There are only so many original things you can say to a bereaved person, only so many ways that you can commiserate without drowning in a sea of clichés.

Most people, quite naturally, grow weary of saying the same thing, or trying to find a new way of saying the same thing. Or they just lose a sense of what you're going through and drift away. Partly because they have their own lives to consider, partly because they are exhausted by trying to understand it. It doesn't make them bad people, or failed people or people somehow lacking in sensitive human spirit. It makes them normal. For who *could* understand such a thing, looking in from outside? Bereavement is impossible to comprehend unless you've been through it or are going through it, and even then it's baffling for most of the time. It is an alien, weird, parallel world, with its own rhythms and strange patterns. It moves slowly. It suffocates. It is relentless. It isolates the people under its spell from the rest of the community. It is contrary, screwed up, a complicated business, so dense, so unpredictable that the greatest minds in the world would struggle with its seeming lack of logic.

And it is full of contradictions. If I just try to answer accurately a simple question, such as 'How am I coping three months on?' my response shows the kind of maddening, confusing, spider's web it weaves.

Okay. I'm coping okay. Well, sort of. But only a little, not a lot. And sometimes. Not always. Occasionally. No, more than that. A fair bit. Though not at all on a bad day or in a bad hour. In a bad hour I'm a terrible, awful, blubbering, helpless, hopeless mess. But, then, I'm also, *sort of*, all right at the same time. I still live. I still function. I still watch the TV, read the paper, laugh and have arguments. I still get cross at things that don't matter, feel frustrations, occasional enjoyment, even the odd thrill. I still have the capacity to feel normal. But if I catch myself feeling normal, I feel guilty that I feel normal so I start feeling terrible again. *Is that clear?*

Just as complex are the stages of grief. When people talk about the pattern of denial, anger, bargaining, depression and acceptance, they don't tell you that those things can all happen in the space of an hour. And start again in a different order. And repeat themselves. Round and round and upside down. Until your head throbs and your eyes hurt and all you want to do is just put your grief down and walk away.

Except you can't.

I tried some bereavement counselling in the aftermath of Vikki's death, to try and sort out some of this confusion in those first few, numbing, scary weeks, when I felt myself stumbling around.

I went to a ramshackle Georgian house behind a tube station in London. There, a woman in her sixties opened the door and led me up three flights of stairs to a room with paint peeling off the walls, a grey-black carpet, a faded geranium in the corner and two large armchairs facing each other. A clipboard lay on one chair. The other was empty but an enormous box of tissues sat next to it. She asked me what I wanted from the sessions.

'I think what I'm looking for is . . . some sort of . . . expert . . . insight . . . or . . . er . . . support to help me through the whole grief process,' I said.

'The first thing I'd say is that I strongly believe there is no grief process.'

This was going to be trickier than I'd thought.

She continued, 'A "process" implies there is a set

series of things that you go through in order to emerge the other side and I don't think grief is quite like that.'

'Okay.' I took a deep breath. 'I think I meant I wanted someone to give me a "map" of some sort.'

'I don't think there is a map.'

'Or at least help me understand.'

'That's implying it's understandable,' she added.

I looked intently at her. She appeared as weary and exhausted as I felt, the endless stories of bereavement, pain and loss etched into her face, recorded in her dry, weathered skin, the heavy lines around her eyes, her unkempt, forgotten hair.

'I just wanted someone . . . . to be a fellow traveller on this . . . er, *path*,' I said.

She looked dubious.

'Highway,' I corrected myself.

'Sounds like a path,' she said.

There was a pause while I racked my brains.

'I'm not trying to be facetious,' she said, 'but you're still making it sound like something you can grasp. Something that's understandable. Maybe none of us can understand it. Maybe it all just happens. And knowing that is the key to getting through it. Do you see what I'm driving at?'

It took me a while but I think I got there eventually. You can't manage your bereavement. It manages you. You just have to sit back and accept it, go with wherever it takes you and try and be philosophical when you find yourself in dark and unpredictable places because if there is one thing that is sure, it is that you have no idea where you are going.

Grief is a rollercoaster full of twists and turns that you go on every day. And every day it's as if they've changed the track. You don't know what's coming. You don't know what's around the corner. You're just trying to hang on, to still be there at the end.

Still being there for a bereaved person is the equivalent of winning the Booker, an Oscar *and* a knighthood. Still being there is such a bloody achievement. Just to get to the end of each bereaved day when you've faced down despair, felt the temptation to crumble, endured guilt, horror, loneliness, regret, guilt again, anguish, frustration and depression. Just to have survived another day, reasonably intact, heart still beating, sanity preserved under the most ferocious assault you've ever dreamed of. Just to be there is everything.

Three months on and I'm still there. I make lists every day in a large hardback book. I walk very fast between appointments, head down. I drink exactly two cans of beer every evening. I sleep so heavily that I wake with a headache.

The shock has subsided – the physical rush that accompanies death has gone. The nights when you lie awake for ever as adrenaline courses round your body, like electricity, and you twitch and flick your fingers and shake your leg and your eyelids wag furiously. The nights when you feel like you're going to explode so you keep moving, trying to calm the raging torrent inside – that rush of anguish and fury and fear that burns as it races round inside your veins and threatens to engulf you.

Something else has replaced it – something constant and nagging, not chronic but constant nonetheless. An ache, a real ache. The dizziness, the tightness, is now a long, slow pull in the pit of the stomach. And where I previously felt like eating very little, now I'm ravenously hungry.

Three months on, and for myself and my little girl there is just the quiet and Vikki's absence to contemplate: the empty side of the bed, the empty chair in the living room, the empty place at dinner when all you can hear is the echo of your own cutlery. And every possession of hers is priceless – every postcard, every Post-it note, every shopping list, every signature, every initial, every tissue found in a coat pocket is significant. Every moment of that person captured, every trace, every smell, every last drop of them. One night I rummage through a bin for hours when I think I've accidentally thrown away a receipt for a railway ticket that wasn't even hers but has her scrawl in the corner.

I make a first attempt to start to rationalise things too, but it's virtually impossible. When I pick up a folder of hers marked 'Holiday' and touch something inside, I start to shake. Everything has this charge. This pulse. This sense of her.

I try to keep a diary, thinking I'll be able to see how I'm progressing. I write a few lines to describe the day's events and add 'BD' or 'GD' at the end. BD for bad day. GD for good. I quickly notice that the entries are very similar and the GDs are few and far between so I stop the diary quickly.

There is so much to do now. As well as the most vital business of looking after my daughter I still face a mountain of admin. There are accounts to be shut, money transferred, debit and credit cards to be stopped, letters to be written. I attack the business of probate just as I'm attacking everything: with a maniacal zeal. I photocopy, get countersignatures, fill in huge forms that take all day. There are piles of paper on the floor, colour-coded lists, charts. Always, there is the Kafkaesque nightmare of institutions to deal with. One day I attempt to close a building society account she held.

'I want to close an account on behalf of my wife who has just died.'

'Okay, sir. I'll put you through, and may I say how sorry I am to hear of your loss.'

'Thank you.'

There is a pause. From the other end of the phone comes very maudlin violin music. It stops abruptly and another voice is on the line. 'Hello, sir. I understand you want to close an account?'

'Yes, on behalf of my wife who has just died.'

'Can I start off by saying how sorry I am for your loss.'

'Thank you.'

'The person you want to talk to is actually on the other line.'

'Right.'

'They'll be with you in a few minutes.'

There is a slightly longer pause and slightly more of the violin music, which seems to have become slightly more maudlin. It stops eventually and another person comes on the line.

'Hello, sir. I understand that you wanted to close an account on behalf of your late wife?'

'That's right.'

'I'll just open a file.'

There is a pause and the music is back – it sounds as if an entire orchestra is weeping. Still, at least I haven't had to hear that he's sorry for my loss.

The music suddenly stops.

'And, by the way, may I say how sorry I am for your loss,' he says.

On another occasion the bland corporate sympathy is replaced by a bizarre lack of understanding.

'I want to close an account that's in my wife's name.'

I am talking to a bored-sounding voice at a bank. It has already taken me nearly ten minutes to get someone on the line. There isn't any funereal music to cover the wait at this place.

'We would need to speak to her,' says the bored voice.

'You can't,' I reply.

'Well, I'm sorry, sir, we won't be able to close it unless we speak to her.'

'But you can't.'

'Why not?'

'She's dead.'

There is a long pause and the voice returns, as defiant as before, 'Well, we still need to speak to her.'

At another building society the lack of understanding has been replaced by bloody-minded bureaucracy. One day I ring them up.

'I'm trying to close an account in the name of my late wife and there seems to be a problem.'

'We need a copy of the death certificate.'

'I sent you a copy of the death certificate three weeks ago.'

'No, you sent us a copy of a copy. We need a copy of the original.'

'What's the difference between a copy and a copy of a copy?'

'It's one more copy.'

'I know that. But if it's a copy anyway, surely it doesn't matter if it's a copy or a copy of a copy.'

'We just need a copy.'

'But I've given you a copy.'

'But it's a copy of a copy. We need a copy of the original.'

'I don't have an original. That's in Hong Kong where she died.'

'Couldn't you get a copy of that?'

'I have got a copy of that! That's what I made a copy of.'

'Of course. Sorry, I'm getting confused. Couldn't you send us the original?'

'The original one in Hong Kong or the original copy?'

'The original copy.'

'No.'

'Why?'

'If I do that, what am I going to make a copy of?'

There is the sound of muffled voices from the other end of the phone.

'A copy of a copy is fine.'

9

THE GREATEST GAME

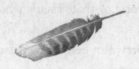

We are in a limo stocked with champagne and we are on our way to Wembley.

This is Vikki's way of preparing for chemotherapy: hiring a mobile bar on wheels and going to the footie. Typical her – defiant, grabbing every opportunity, enthusiastic, borderline eccentric. Refusing to give in. And her way again. Her way.

Mind you, this is no ordinary game. This is no stopgap distraction. Some meaningless little football match that enchants only the diehards, of no consequence, nothing at stake, nothing to tell your grandchildren about.

The game we're going to is the game. The one that determines who will be promoted to the Premiership – the richest game in the world, as everyone calls it. Charlton versus Sunderland.

Charlton are our adopted team, the local team. We got involved through an old friend who encouraged us to come *along. Their ground is across the park from where we live, in Greenwich. We can leave at two-fifteen, grab the train and still be in our seats for kick-off at three. Through Maze Hill, Westcombe Park, then off at Charlton station, up the steps and down Floyd Road, past the chip shop to the ground, hidden within the network of Victorian terraced houses.*

Vikki and I have other teams, other long-term loves, Leeds in her case, Brighton and Hove Albion in mine, but somehow we've just got attached to Charlton. They're a new friend and we can't help liking them. There's something about Charlton. Unfashionable underdogs, salt of the earth, the very opposite of flashy. Real. Honest. Sound too: they're always winning Community Club of the Year. At one stage they even formed a political party in the local elections in a bid to be allowed back to their spiritual home in the borough. Years of bad financial management by previous regimes had left them groundless and on the brink of bankruptcy. Slowly we've been drawn in. We started off watching the odd match, and before long we were buying season tickets. We got hooked.

If you'd asked me before whether it was possible to get emotionally involved with a football team other than your own I'd have said no . . . until Charlton came along. Slowly they've wiggled their way into our affections and we've become buddies – not lovers: that's Leeds for Vikki and Brighton for me. That heart-stopping visceral connection never changes. But everyone is allowed friends as well. And Charlton are definitely that. Strong, reliable friends. Now they're at Wembley, on the brink of something momentous. And we are too.

Chemotherapy is the big unknown. It's the start of a regime that will last several months, a long, complex assault course with an uncertain end. Vikki is booked to go into the hospital for her first round on the Tuesday and the game is the day before.

In my ignorance I didn't really know what chemotherapy was – I thought it was just some giant machine zapping electric currents at the cancer. I didn't know it meant people in chairs quietly having drugs. But that is what it is. One person in a room or sometimes whole lines of patients in a chemotherapy suite hooked up to drips while specially trained nurses very slowly inject highly specialised, highly toxic drugs into their systems. Drugs that flatten everything inside the human body, including, hopefully, the cancer cells. Indiscriminate bombing, total destruction, the kind you welcome if you've been diagnosed.

And while this is happening, while the war is being waged, the patients read magazines or listen to music through headphones. Sometimes they chat gently to the nurses or peer out of the window or doze. It's a strange meeting of the normal and the abnormal. A life-altering process shrouded in mundanity. Like open-heart surgery done in the local library.

Then when the chemotherapy drugs have been administered, along with the anti-sickness ones that accompany them, the patient is free to leave, after a suitably British cup of hospital tea with biscuits, invariably pleased and relieved, mentally checking off this part of their cycle as they go. Everyone's course of chemo is different, calculated according to the type of cancer, the stage of the disease, even the weight of the individual. But everyone is equally desperate to get to the end of it.

The first time you have the drugs, they want you to stay in hospital overnight just in case you react badly, sickness being one of the many side effects. There are so many others it takes them a good hour to tell us and we still leave our pre-meeting clutching information sheets. Apparently your hair falls out, your nails crack, you can get dizzy, depressed, swollen legs, painful joints; you can gain weight, lose weight; you can lose your sense of taste. The list is endless. Of course, you may not get any of these. Maybe you'll be fine.

So, we go to a football match in a limo, in those last sticky-slow hours, to try to forget all of that – the nails and the hair and the sickness. We go to try to be normal for just a little longer.

The game kicks off, in that vast bowl that is old Wembley, its 76,000 seats filled to capacity. In that moment it is impossible to believe in ill-health or chemo. There's just the game. Only the game. And the noise. The crowd. That in itself is good.

And what a game it is. Charlton go ahead early, and the stand explodes, and Vikki is jumping up and down, and we are transported on a wave of delirium. Sunderland equalise, and we sink horribly. Then Sunderland go ahead again before we've even had time to absorb the disappointment of their first goal, and while their first was a shock we're now empty, losing hope. There are misses and close calls, a pass that nearly makes it, a shot that is just blocked at the last moment. Then, all too soon, the referee is blowing his whistle for half-time, and we slump in our seats, shoulders hunched, bleary-eyed, shattered and thrilled by what we've just seen.

For the next fifteen minutes we babble away excitedly, reflecting on the game, and only from time to time do I see in her eyes that faraway look as she remembers other, more serious things, but for the most part we're just swept away by the sheer screaming brilliance of it all.

The players reappear and the whole exhausting drama starts up again.

Charlton come storming out and equalise, but Sunderland go ahead again. We're beside ourselves when Charlton equalise a third time. What fighting spirit. What resource. I catch Vikki's eye again and we both smile.

Extra time arrives, and in the searing heat the players are wilting, the crowd too, our nerves tweaked, twisted and torn off. It all looks lost as Sunderland go ahead yet again, and with the score at 4–3, time is ticking by. Everyone around us is tense. Some worried faces are permanently framed by hands. Other people constantly look at their watches.

The ball comes across – rifled at great speed by Charlton's Jones into the Sunderland penalty area. One last attempt. One last chance. It's aimed at Mendonca, the Charlton striker, but is slightly behind him. It's far too hard for him to control. Surely only a genius would get that, not a Charlton player. But he just manages to catch the ball on the tip of his outstretched right foot and flicks it up before swivelling and, in one superb graceful movement, volleying the ball into the Sunderland net. Charlton have equalised and, from the depths of despair, a seemingly hopeless position has been rescued: 4–4. Minutes later and the final whistle blows.

I look at Vikki. Now we just shake our heads. It almost feels as if the game is following some pre-determined script, especially for us.

Penalties next and even more drama. Penalties – the most gut-wrenching heart-stopping denouement possible. One kick that decides the future of players, fans, clubs. Of money, hopes, dreams. Just one kick.

As the players gather in the centre of the pitch to prepare I find myself thinking of those other things now, of the harsh reality that faces us the next day, and then I realise I haven't been thinking of that at all in this cauldron of excitement. I look across at Vikki and wonder if it isn't the same for her – if that grim contemplation hasn't been utterly chased away, if only for a few delicious, thrilling moments.

'Some game,' I say.

'Fantastic,' she agrees. And she beams from ear to ear.

Then the whistle blows and the whole insane rollercoaster sets off again.

As a Charlton player slowly walks to the penalty area and puts the ball down, Vikki has her hands over her face and is staring through her fingers – he scores. So do the

Sunderland player and the Charlton player after him and the Sunderland player after him and the Charlton player again . . .

And on and on it goes.

It is 5–5 and sudden death. Everything moves up a notch. It's 6–5, then 6–6, and people around us can't watch at all. They've turned their backs now – and on the pitch, Christ, it's Charlton's Sean Newton and he can barely walk he's so nervous. Why is he taking one? He never takes penalties! And people in the crowd are clasping each other, burying their heads in each other's shoulders, and all of us, all of us, are just wrung out with the tension, clinging on. Newton steps up and hits the ball and it is to the goalkeeper's left, exactly where he is diving, and for a split second it looks as if Perez, for Sunderland, must reach it but Newton's penalty is just high enough: he lifts it over the goalkeeper's right hand and we all breathe again, before gathering ourselves for the next. I have a vision of this going on forever – this exquisite torture, this heart-stopping rhythm of rising tension and release. Now it's Michael Gray from Sunderland and he's measuring his run up and wait, it's a bit short, isn't it? I look at Vikki and squeeze her arm, and I know that none of her, absolutely none of her, is thinking of the cancer. All of her is just taken with the moment, with this penalty in this football match. This stupid, meaningless football match.

This fantastic life-changing football match.

Gray is standing, ready to go, hands on hips, and the

referee blows his whistle. He steps up and . . . I don't quite see what happens at first because Vikki is all over me, jumping madly, and the people in front are jumping up and down too, and an old man below us loses his glasses and literally gets swallowed by the crowd as he leans forward and seems to disappear behind a curtain of flailing legs and feet, then emerges with the glasses forlorn and broken in his hand. But with a massive smile on his face.

Gray has missed.

Charlton have won.

CHARLTON HAVE WON!!!

All the fear and terror and shock of the last few weeks seem concentrated into this one moment and are then released, as if they've been lit by a match and blown into the air with a resounding *BANG*.

All around, adults, like children stamping in ecstasy when they get their Christmas presents, are shouting and screaming, flowing back and forth on the steps of crumbling old Wembley.

I'm shouting at Vikki: 'It's a sign! It's a sign! See? Do you see it?' Like a mad person.

And for that brief moment, I absolutely believe what I'm saying.

It IS a sign: Vikki is going to win. Just like Charlton. She's going to win against all the odds. She's going to be fine. And the ecstasy of it all sweeps us up in its grasp and carries us away, a massive surge of adrenaline. Sure. Indestructible. Then we hug each other almost too tight and in that moment I feel that we are powerful, we are irresistible.

Vikki is going to win.

Twenty-four hours later she is sitting in a room at the hospital. Her left arm is hooked up to a saline drip. With her left hand she holds a large glass of water with ice that she sips from. Her chemo nurse is slowly pumping the chemicals into her vein, holding a syringe in the cannula on her right hand and squeezing the end of the syringe so slowly, so gradually, that it is barely perceptible. I sit and watch from across the room in a chair. The only sounds are muffled voices from the corridor and the occasional rattle of ice on Vikki's teeth as she swills the water round her mouth, holding it there for as long as possible – it helps to ward off dryness and mouth sores. The stillness is in total contrast to the previous day when we were joyfully rampaging about like excited apes.

The nurse is on the last drug of the three she has to administer. They all have separate functions and work differently in combination. Vikki's regime involves her having six courses of chemotherapy. On the first, third and fifth cycles she is to have three drugs, on the others just two.

The chemo drugs are often violent colours, as if cockily declaring their own shocking nature. This last one is ruby red. As the nurse finishes she takes the syringe out of the cannula on Vikki's hand, carefully places it on the tray with the other syringes, then stands and peels off her gloves. 'Well done,' she says. 'That's chemo number one finished.'

As she leaves the room to let us relax, we switch on the TV and see Charlton parading the trophy they won the day before. They are driving through south-east London and it is a typical Charlton affair – the opposite of glamorous, rain lashing down on the players as they huddle on the roof of an open-top bus. But we don't notice the rain.

Vikki isn't sick in the night. Not even remotely. And she doesn't faint or swell or suffer any of the symptoms we'd been warned about.

And to all those people who say football isn't important and doesn't carry an almost magical significance: you couldn't be more wrong. Not only have Charlton won, it feels like we have too.

10

THE DANCE

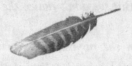

'Hey, good to see you.'

'Good to see you too.'

'It's been a while . . .'

The young commissioning editor looks at me as I sit opposite him and his assistant. He has a smile fixed to his face. It's a TV kind of smile, which isn't surprising because this is TV. It's a confident, practised smile but it doesn't mean anything.

We're in a modern glass office. From here you can see a larger open-plan space that stretches out for some distance and is mostly populated by people in their twenties wearing T-shirts and jeans.

I'm back at work. I have to be back at work. I'm self-employed. No work means no money, but it's good too: it acts as an escape, a chance to throw off the mental chains – just for a few hours. To get in touch with another world that isn't full of death and grieving.

I'm here to pitch new ideas – three, in fact. I'll pitch them and, with luck, the TV channel will get enthused about one. They may commission a script or a treatment of the idea. They may also ask me to go away and rethink one of them.

Of course, they may just reject the whole lot.

Yet as we sit down I'm feeling confident. This is familiar territory. The glass office. The pitch meeting. The TV people across the table. I've done it dozens of times before in dozens of offices a little like this.

'So what are you up to?' the commissioning editor says, looking at me.

The TV smile is still there and I like that smile because I know that smile. I know where it leads, what will happen now.

What will happen is that I will take the floor and outline the various other projects I have on the go with other TV channels, other commissioning editors, all of which I will describe in a positive, enthusiastic fashion. I will make them sound exciting and current, as though they're happening imminently, if they aren't already underway. I will talk of casting and use the word 'production' a lot, even if they haven't yet had a green light. I will be slick and amusing, professional and irreverent. It will make me look interesting, relevant and desirable, just the sort of writer the commissioning editor wants to be in business with. After I've finished, there will be a kind of glow in the room, and the commissioning editor and his assistant will be primed and ready to buy my new ideas. Even if they don't, I'll leave the room still looking credible, a strong contender the next time I return.

So this tiny casual preamble matters. It is important. I am not a 'name' writer. I can't rely on them coming to me, blinded by my reputation, their hands outstretched for gifts. I've had a cult hit a while back. I am, I think, fairly well regarded within the industry. People will know my name. I'm no journeyman. I'm no hack. But I'm not a star either. So every time, in every meeting, when we get to the inevitable question – 'So what are you up to?' – it's a moment of significance.

I have to perform. I don't have a choice. It's the way it is. This is TV.

This is *the dance*.

All writers, apart from the superstars, have to do that dance – to learn the art of the first ten minutes. The first ten minutes, which have so little to do with the rest of the meeting yet at the same time have everything to do with it.

I can do it pretty well. I learned when I was young about the importance of selling – my dad worked in advertising and would regale us round the dinner table with tales of successful campaigns for Potterton boilers, Swedish breathing equipment, revolutionary seed drills and ornate smokeless candles with funky designs on the outside. He would talk about the 'art' of the sell, about communication, about fixing someone with your eyes, pointing out the words and making them feel that all they wanted to do was buy what you had to offer.

I've been burnishing my skills ever since. Sounding upbeat, glass half full. Positive. Talking about possibilities, potential. Weaving an interesting tale. Painting vivid pictures in the air. Learning how to drop a name skilfully so it doesn't sound a clang when it lands.

I've had a lot of practice and I've honed my craft. Through experience, I know what goes down well. I have refined my technique through countless meetings and can turn it on and off like a tap. I can be down, feeling grumpy and negative, and yet, when I get into TV Land, instantly transform into someone bright and optimistic. I can create a good atmosphere. I can sparkle.

I can *do the dance* pretty well.

And, what's more, even if I can't, I can fake it: sometimes there's little happening in your career – projects have stalled, been forgotten, fallen away, series have been cancelled. Sometimes there's very little to shout about. Sometimes there's almost nothing you can dredge up to make yourself look good. Or impressive. Or promising. Or just average.

That's when I improvise, tweak or, as a fellow writer once said with a mixture of disbelief and admiration, 'rustle up something from the bullshit files'.

That's when I manage to spin my way out of a dire situation with a neat little shuffle, a side-step, sleight of hand, perhaps saying a project is still in play when I know it's going down the tubes or that a pilot is going to series when I know very well it'll never go ahead unless the channel controller gets a sense of humour transplant.

I'm also pretty good at finding one of those meaningless phrases that just sounds impressive in the room.

Example one, said with a sombre expression: 'I have a LOT of interest in the US in my pilot.'

Example two, accompanied by a nonchalant sweep of a hand through the hair: 'I'm talking to Sky about a comedy drama.'

Example three, said with quiet intensity, as if I've just discovered Tutankhamun's holiday home: 'I'm actually working on a couple of things for Steve Coogan's Company,' which probably means I'm going to give the projects to them when they've been written, at which point they will turn them down.

Lately, for the first time, I've been feeling a little less bullish, a little less confident about the whole idea of work, of putting myself out there, meeting people, pitching to them, exposing my ideas to the possibility of rejection. It hasn't been a constant feeling but a slow-burning doubt that suddenly flares and retreats but never completely disappears. On occasion, I've felt uneasy. Edgy, even fearful. Certainly unsure. I've put it down to nerves. I haven't done this in a while and the day-to-day involvement, where you get into a certain rhythm, where you get battle-hardened, inured to the possibility of defeat, is a distant memory. Sometimes it's hard to picture my old confident self, bouncing from one meeting to the next. I know I was that person. It's just sometimes I can't quite feel it.

Then there are the extraordinary events of the last few years and months. All that turmoil, that stomach-churning, adrenaline-fuelled lurching from medical crisis to medical crisis, that emotional fury, that hellish noise. All I have craved for a while is peace and withdrawal, a restorative calm. Suddenly the TV world seems a loud, unsettling and unpredictable place.

And I've had enough surprises.

Still, I've convinced myself that once I'm in the meeting, in the full glare of the lights, back in the old routine, it will all come back. I've just been away for a bit, that's all. Give me five minutes. Let me crack the first joke. I'll relax into it. You never lose it, do you? It's just like riding a bike.

It will all come back again. It must come back. It *will* come back.

'Busy, then?'

The smile is still there. The commissioning editor is watching me. As is his assistant. The moment is here, undoubtedly. There is no putting it off. So I smile back, gather myself, draw a deep breath, look out and . . . and . . . and . . .

Nothing.

Nothing.

Absolutely nothing.

Nothing comes out of my mouth.

Nothing is in my head.

Nothing.

And I'm aware of something else. A kind of suspension, a sense of gliding, floating. A feeling of not being rooted, not being solid, not being there at all. Like a hot-air balloon drifting smoothly, inexorably, away from its mooring. I'm feeling a very strange detachment.

Instinctively part of me reaches out, trying to find the stake to which I was tied, but I'm reaching into nothing. I know what I want to do. I want to answer him but the words won't come.

And suddenly the dance seems puzzling and unfamiliar, as if I've never done it before. A strange new set of steps with different rhythms played out over unfamiliar music.

'Er . . .' I stumble. I can feel my cheeks getting hot. My back is sweating through my shirt. I feel uncomfortable. There's no brightness, no energy. I can't summon it up. And, worse, I can't fake it.

I'm not even really panicking. If I was it would give me an edge. But I have . . . nothing.

Just then the conversation switches as a young PA interrupts us with an important message for the commissioning editor, and soon the others are talking and I'm looking on. They're like shapes behind a gauze. Just outlines. Muffled and distant.

Then it comes to me. The reason for the sweats and the silence and the torpor and the floating: *I just don't care about this anymore.*

There have been signs, warnings. A week before I was on a train heading into London from Norfolk and a thought flashed into my head, prompted by the crowded streets, flooded with people scurrying to work. A thought I had never really contemplated. *Maybe I should do something else.* Something other than writing.

That has never happened before. Never, in the previous twenty-three years of head-down commitment, has that thought ever occurred. It has never so much as popped up casually. Never appeared as a distant dot on the horizon.

Something other than writing. But what?

My proper work CV reads like a bad sitcom. I did a week's gooseberry-picking in 1981 and spent four days selling word processors that same summer holiday. (Not that I sold any. I was completely ignorant about technology at the time, and if someone came into the shop and said, 'Do you have a Commodore PET?' I would say, 'I'll see,' then go into a back room, shut the door, count to fifty, come out, and say, 'No'.)

A week's gooseberry-picking and four days not selling word processors. Throw in some desultory gardening, when I destroyed my client's tomato plants, and that's pretty much it in the way of having a normal job. The rest of the time I'd spent writing and prancing around various stages. I don't have much in the way of experience. Maybe I could retrain.

I briefly consider thoughts of teaching, of being some inspirational guru-like figure, espousing great works of literature, jumping on tables to rapturous applause. The thought appeals, the idea of inspiring a generation, kick-starting the careers of at least one Man Booker Prize winner who, in a future profile in *The Times*, will quote me as a seminal influence.

But I think too of the staffroom politics, the uninterested kids, the philistine parents, the targets I'll have to meet, the exam-factory mentality. And I wouldn't be allowed to climb on tables for health and safety reasons.

Then I consider being a musician. This is obviously something I've done intermittently before. There was *that* gig, of course, when I saw Vikki, but there were many others; the teenage residency in the nightclub outside Brighton; later, jazz and poetry at the Purcell Room on the South Bank; a spot at the Fulham Greyhound pub in London; a gig supporting Squeeze at the Town and Country Club. I played on some jingles, a couple of commercials, some TV theme tunes, some live TV shows. There was even an eccentric tour of Scotland, which included a riotous gig at a pyramid sales conference (now they *really* like getting on tables) and an evening at a fearsome Trawler-men's ball, where they put bottles of whisky on each table instead of wine. All great fun. It's what I enjoy.

But do I really want to travel the length and breadth of the country gigging, away from my daughter? Who would look after her?

Do I really want to live such unsociable hours? Trundling up and down the M11 getting back at four in the morning? Because that is what it would mean. There are only so many properly paid gigs in Norfolk, only so many weddings and birthday parties each weekend.

Do I really want to be a nomad at the age of forty-four? Stuck in a van for hours a day with a bunch of people I barely know?

As Charlie Watts once said, of playing with the Stones, for every five years of work, there's twenty years' hanging around. And he gets to hang around in a limo, not a Ford Transit.

'So, come on then – spill!'

Back in the office the PA has departed and the commissioning editor is looking at me again, hopefully. With that smile.

I have one last shot. Maybe this time I'll wake up. Maybe the old Carl will appear.

He *must*. Because it's me now, just me. On my own. I am the only breadwinner now Vikki is gone, the only one to bring the money in. I must get a commission.

So what if I don't care about it any more? It doesn't matter. I just have to do it. For my daughter's sake as well as mine.

For a second the clouds seem to clear. Suddenly my brain is thinking work thoughts and I'm aware of the other scripts I'm writing at the moment. It's not that I haven't been productive. I have. Vikki's death has been the spur for all kinds of projects.

It's all coming back now . . .

There's a bereavement diary I am thinking about turning into a book, a new sitcom about a man establishing his life after the death of his wife, an idea for a comedy drama series set at various funerals.

I am the king of grief, the go-to man for misery. I feel it. I think it. I write it. It's coming out of every pore, bleeding out of every vein. I have pages of the stuff.

And yet . . .

All of these projects are at an early stage, they aren't finished, they haven't been pitched. There are no glamorous names attached; they are not exciting or current. They don't yet have the wow factor. What's more, feeling as I do, leaden and slow-witted, I realise I can't disguise that. I can't shine them up for public consumption, pimp them to make them look more than they are. I just can't do it.

'Something exciting, I'll bet,' says the assistant, hopefully. I try to smile.

The commissioning editor and the assistant reach

across the table, mouths open, expecting more. I summon every bit of half-remembered enthusiasm. I clear my throat. 'Obviously . . . er . . . a couple of things,' I say hesitantly.

There. I've started. Phew. Instinct has finally kicked in and, from the deepest, darkest recess, some reflex has bounced me back into the game.

'Great!' says the commissioning editor, leaning further forward. He wants more.

They look at me. Willing me to lace up my dancing shoes one more time.

'There's a sitcom I'm working on.' That's more like it, I tell myself.

'Sounds interesting,' says the assistant.

See? He certainly thinks so.

'A series?' asks the commissioning editor.

'Pilot,' I correct him. *Whoops. You didn't need to say that. You could have left it more open.*

'When's it being shown?' asks the assistant.

'It's only in development,' I add. *Don't tell them that! That just sounds negative. And don't say 'only' in development. It's in development. That in itself is pretty damn good. Sound excited, for Christ's sake! Have you forgotten everything you've learned in TV?*

I look across the table. Despite my attempts at gentle self-destruction, they're still there, the commissioning editor and his assistant. They look expectant. I can feel their hands outstretched. They're inviting me in.

This is the moment, I say to myself, your best and final chance. Go for it! You've done this before. If you can't do it properly, just fake it. Make something up. Pretend. Lie. This is TV.

'Anything else, apart from the pilot?' says the assistant.

I open my mouth, hoping that, like some slavering Pavlovian dog, I will react automatically and, without thought or planning, pluck something from obscurity and hurl it like a fireball onto the table.

I lick my lips. My mouth is dry. 'I'm off on holiday soon,' I say, defeated.

There's a silence. They look disappointed. I feel I've crossed some invisible line. As if something in my professional life, the life I pursued fanatically for almost a quarter of a century, has changed forever.

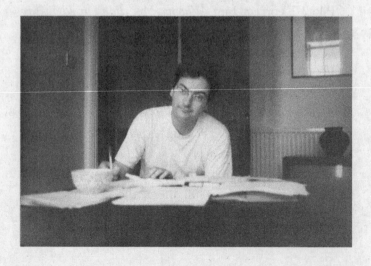

II

UNKIND WORDS

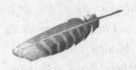

'Why are we out walking in this heat?'

I can hear the irritation in my voice and we've barely started along the path.

It's a late September morning in the mid-1990s. Back, way back, before cancer. Before the fear and worry and darkness descend.

Vikki and I have come away for a quick break and are outside a small town in the South of France called Saint-Paul-de-Vence, a stunning cluster of stone houses wrapped within a medieval wall, a picture-perfect dream, up the winding road from Nice.

At the gated entrance to the town wall there's a glorious square shaded by trees where the old men play boules and drinks are brought out with great ceremony on trays to be drunk at the surrounding tables. To the left is the famous Colombe d'Or hotel where artists paid for their stay by *donating pictures – you have to be careful in the dining room with your pasta sauce in case you flick it onto the Braque on the wall behind you. In the shimmering late-summer sun, as we look back down on the square and the shadows of the leaves that dance on the backs of the people and the beige sandy surface of the ground, it's a beautiful sight. But right now I'm not appreciating it. I'm not appreciating anything's beauty.*

'How much further?' I ask grumpily.

'Just over this little rise,' she replies cheerfully.

We are climbing up a steep, dusty track, Vikki in front, then me. We're across the road from the village's entrance and we're heading for the white gallery, the Fondation Maeght, that sits on the hill above the town. It's about ten in the morning and you can hear the cicadas buzzing.

It is hot. Very hot.

'Do we really have to do this? You keep organising these day trips and . . .'

She looks down at me from her elevated position on the path above, defiantly smiling. 'Oh, come on! You'll enjoy it when you get there.'

'I won't.'

You can hear the irritation in my voice, not helped by the fact that I have already bashed my head on a metal Alexander Calder sculpture beside the pool in the Colombe d'Or as we nipped in to have a look round.

She turns away from me and strides ahead once more.

She has organised this trip as she has organised all our

trips – immaculately, squeezing the maximum out of the adventure. She has the guide books, the maps, we have an itinerary: the Matisse church down the road; the art gallery up the hill; the markets in Nice; a bus trip to Grasse. No one could have done it better, more thoroughly. And in my crabby, cranky current mood I couldn't give a damn.

'Oh God,' I mutter, as we reach the top of the rise only to find another length of path stretching out ahead. I can feel the sun baking my arms and neck. I can feel the weight of my rucksack containing the exquisite picnic lunch she has already prepared. All I can see up ahead is a steep path that seems to wind endlessly into the hills.

'Oh come on, Ern. You'll survive.'

This is a playful nickname, an ironic reference to my profession in the comedy business and my apparent kinship with the unfunny one from the very funny duo. Usually it makes me smile but something about her using it now just makes me more annoyed. 'This is supposed to be a holiday!' I say.

She doesn't look back as she continues up.

I pause momentarily and look at her, determinedly striding off up the hill.

Another couple are descending along the same path.

'Come on,' she says, without looking back. 'I think I can see the top.'

I sigh and try to move off again, grudgingly, but this time something in me refuses and I find myself rooted. I can feel something new now, something different, far off, a distant roar getting nearer and nearer, a new energy that is suddenly flowing through me. A sharp, spiteful energy that causes my muscles to tighten and my arms and feet to lock, as they try to contain this force, this rush of pure, foaming anger.

And I'm aware, at that moment, that my body is going nowhere. It is adamant. Intractable. Set like concrete.

She turns once more.

'Come on,*' she says, imploring.*

I don't move.

'It'll be like a lot of things. You'll be glad when you've done it,' she says.

But I'm way beyond that point now. My jaw is clenched and I'm shaking, and what comes out from me is part scream, part hiss, part furious, raging psychotic roar.

'I FUCKING HATE ART GALLERIES, OKAY?'

The words are way angrier than even I intend, each syllable hard and physical as it's hurled in her direction. My throat seems to twist around each sound as I spit it out and the rest of my body tightens with it. My face is puckered and puce with exhaustion and frustration, and at that moment whatever I feel doesn't much resemble love.

She looks shocked.

I'm just as startled at what has come out – that voice didn't even sound like mine.

And I don't hate art galleries. I'm just lashing out. Yet still its cruel edge, its sharpness, surprises me.

For a second we stand there motionless and awkward.

The people ahead of us pass us on the way down. They

don't look at us and I'm sure they must have heard.

I look away briefly, back down the dusty track. I need a second to compose myself. And I want to hide my embarrassment.

When I turn back to Vikki, I notice something has changed in her expression. She looks hurt.

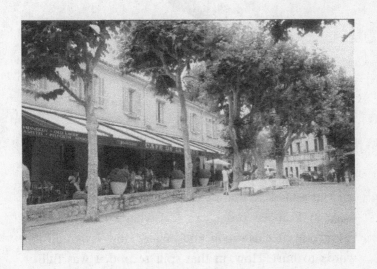

12

NEVER

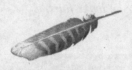

I shudder as the words come back to me now. I can still feel their venom, years later.

It's four months after her death and I can take myself back in a blink to that dusty slope outside the beautiful town in France. And I can feel what I felt then. The rising tide of frustration and anger. How I wanted the words to hurt. How, in that split second, I was full of cruelty. How I wanted her to feel that too.

She had planned the trip so lovingly. She had wanted to share a beautiful moment, looking at beautiful pictures. She wanted me to enjoy the art the way she did. She wanted us to share in something. She wanted us to be happy.

And right then, all I really wanted to do was destroy it all.

But, then, I was tired and hot, and she'd probably tried to pack in a bit too much. Besides, which couple hasn't exchanged bitter, angry words? Everyone does it from time to time, don't they? Even the most loving couples, tempers frayed, hassled, weary, halfway up a hill, lose it with each other.

Which couple hasn't had a moment or two like that? A strange, savage split second eruption, so lacking in love, affection and all the things that are supposed to bind you together. It's just human nature, isn't it? It happens. That's relationships. That's life.

Four months on from her death and I have many negative thoughts. They rush in on me when I'm tired and fragile: at five in the morning when I wake, as I always do, and see the empty side of the bed, hear the silence in the room except for my own breath.

In these dark early days after her going, it seems all the good stuff has been temporarily side lined, squeezed out by the regrets that pour in on me, like a vast swollen river that I haven't a hope of repelling. I worry that I could have, should have, done more with regard to her illness. Even though I went to every appointment, scan and day of treatment with her, I still feel as if I could have done more. Maybe I just didn't ask the right questions at the right time? If I'd taken just a little more notice when the consultant said this or that, could I have made a crucial point that would have made a difference?

Could I have researched more and found some miracle cure that no one else knew about? Did I make her the right food? Could I have created a better living environment? *Could I have saved her?*

And in the midst of these life-and-death questions are the everyday regrets – the small things that happen across the years in any relationship; the odd inevitable unkind word spoken, the missed opportunity, the moment not fully realised, the occasion when I feel I came up short or just wasn't as good as I might have been. The morning I was crabby and unhelpful, the time I could have been more supportive of one of her suggestions, the occasions I could have been a better husband, partner, cheerleader, supporter, friend, the many casual and trivial incidents that in life count for little but in the shadow of death seem to count for so much.

Yet still, strangely, the most persistent regret of all is that outburst halfway up a hill on holiday in France. That one sentence on that one day, with the sun beating down and the rage in my voice and her face caught in a moment of surprise and disappointment.

And hurt.

More than any others that flit across my vision, this memory returns again and again. It refuses to leave me alone. Small in the great scheme of things but massive in what it reveals. Words said then that I can't now undo. Words left hanging.

For that's the point. I can't take them back. I can't explain them. I can't make them better. I can't revisit them in any way. I can't re-examine them. Can't suddenly decide to discuss them, years on. I can't lean across to her in bed and say, with a smile, 'You know that awful time when I yelled at you in France all those years ago? It's been bugging me ever since and I never meant . . .'

I can't say it any more. It's a physical impossibility.

Because she's gone.

And although we moved on from that brief, furious outburst (I gave in and spent a sullen morning wandering around the art gallery and we joked about it later), right now it still feels like unfinished business because the opportunity, the freedom for me to go back to that moment, is gone forever.

I'd still like to be able to revisit it because I'd still like to revisit everything. Or just *know* I can. Every little unkindness, unresolved irritation, crossed wire and misunderstanding. Every misapprehension. Every part of the fabric of my life with her, imperfect and good.

Somehow that exchange halfway up a hill in the South of France has become a symbol of everything I can't do now.

Because she is no longer here. She is just lost to me. And everyone else. She is a terrible silence. She is a past tense. She is gone, never to return.

I will *never* be able to hold her, *never* be able to comfort her, *never* share a joke with her again.

Never be able to discuss shouting at her like a lunatic halfway up a hill in France.

NEVER.

She is a *never*.

And as I feel the finality of that – as soon as I feel the cold draught of that door slamming – I experience a wave of panic, a physical fear. Adrenaline pours through my system and I'm shaking. Trapped. Like a cornered animal.

The words scream out from somewhere deep inside me: PLEASE JUST BRING HER BACK.

But there is no reply.

Because there is no answer.

No solution.

No reassurance.

Just the silence.

But I can't accept it. Not now. Not yet. I can't contemplate it. The thought of never seeing her again. It's too much. Too utterly terrifying.

I have to feel the possibility of reconnecting somewhere, somehow. I have to. It's a necessity. A question of my own survival. For if I don't convince myself I'll see her again, it feels as if I have nothing left. Nothing to help lift me out of this state. Nothing to pull me forwards and onwards.

So I close my eyes and imagine her. The look of her.

The sound of her. Those eyes. And I try to reconnect with that sense of her.

I try to find her, for I cannot, will not, accept that she has become nothing. Become a never.

After the funeral a friend gives me a copy of the famous poem by Henry Holland, Canon of St Paul's, 'Death Is Nothing At All', and I am struck by its words.

After a few weeks, when I start to put away some of the many other cards and letters of condolence in a box, I make a point of leaving it out, giving it a position of some prominence on my bedside table. I'm especially glad of it now. I read it so often the words are soon committed to memory and I find myself reciting it at home, outside, walking on the seashore, driving through a nearby village. It is familiar to the point of cliché, uncomplicated and sentimental, but at an uncertain time, caught between fear and panic, it speaks to me perfectly, offering clarity, comfort and hope. The merest sliver of hope to this beleaguered, struggling individual. The undoubtedly romantic notion of someday, somehow seeing her again.

> Death is nothing at all
> I have only slipped away into the next room.
> I am I and you are you.
> Whatever we were to each other,
> That we still are.

Call me by my old familiar name
Speak to me in the easy way
Which you always used.
Put no difference into your tone.
Wear no forced air of solemnity or sorrow.

Laugh as we always laughed
At the little jokes we enjoyed together.
Play. Smile. Think of me. Pray for me.
Let my name be ever the household word
That it always was.
Let it be spoken without effect.
Without the trace of a shadow on it.

Life means all it ever meant.
It is the same that it ever was.
There is absolute unbroken continuity.
Why should I be out of mind
Because I am out of sight?

I am but waiting for you
For an interval.
Somewhere. Very near.
Just around the corner.

All is well.

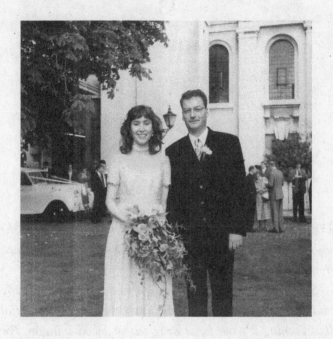

13

READY MADE

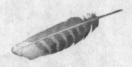

Vikki races down the stairs into the kitchen. 'Hurry,' she says. 'We've got to be there in half an hour.' She is just back from work. I've only been home five minutes.

She is halfway through her first course of chemotherapy and it's going well, but although we're due at the hospital that evening it's not for a drug test or blood infusion. For once, it's something a little more pleasant, a little more edifying, a little more uplifting: a support group meeting.

She takes the two packages out of her plastic carrier bag and plonks them on the kitchen surface. 'Is the oven ready?'

'Nearly,' I reply. I'm looking at my watch, calculating.

She bends down and lifts out two plates from the cupboard. 'Just chuck them in,' she says. The knives and forks rattle as she throws them on top of the plates and then sets about hurriedly cutting some broccoli.

I pull the cardboard sleeves off the packaging and try to peel the film lid off the top of the first lasagne but I'm hurrying so it tears, leaving some little shards of plastic hanging off the sides, and the tips of my fingers coated with food. I start to pull off the shards one by one but my fingers are greasy and the whole container shudders, sending the lasagne up one side so it nearly spills out. I shake it back down so it's level. It's on my other hand as well now and there is a dob of food on my jumper. I quickly attempt to take the lid off the second container but with two greasy hands it is even harder and the same thing happens, only worse; larger, more numerous shards of plastic are left poking out the sides of this one. 'I need some scissors,' I say.

'They look fine. The heat'll kill that stuff,' she says. She grabs both the containers from me and plonks them in the oven. I don't disagree with her as I'm starving. Thursday nights are like this – barely time to get home and eat before the meeting starts. No time to do anything.

The food is supposed to take twenty minutes but I turn up the oven higher and take it out after fifteen. Unfortunately she's put the containers too near the wall of the oven so one has actually stuck to it but with the aid of a fish slice we're able to prise it away. We empty the containers onto the plates and stand at the breakfast bar to eat.

'Come on,' she says.

We pile into the car and race over the hill to the hospital. There is nowhere to park at the front so we drive round and leave the car in one of the staff spaces at the rear of the building. Then we double back, go through the main entrance and down the familiar corridor then left down the stairs and into the basement, past the anaesthetic room, the holding bay and the operating theatre. At the end of the corridor there is a conference room with a woman standing, smiling, in the doorway. She beckons us in. She's wearing a wig and has no eyebrows.

Mary is proud to be the head of the Breast Cancer Support Group. Keeps her going, she says. Keeps her busy. No time to think, which is a good thing – she has been battling the disease herself for a while. A well-dressed, spirited woman she'll never give up. 'Just about to start,' she says enthusiastically.

The conference room has a dark carpet and light blue walls. Anodyne pictures of woodland streams and meadows hang across it at intervals. There are two banks of chairs, which face in the same direction. A projector has been set up, which looks forward onto a large screen. There is barely an empty seat.

The room is full of women of various ages – the youngest in their late twenties, the oldest probably in their sixties. There is one other man apart from myself. About eighty per cent of the women have no eyebrows. Most of them look like they have wigs on too. You can tell because the standard NHS ones are variable in quality and often unfortunately just look like wigs, at odds with the wearer, not well fitted, and harsh unsubtle colours.

Vikki was fortunate and got hers from a theatrical wig-maker. It's properly fitted, made of real human hair woven onto a base. You really couldn't tell it's a wig and it gives her confidence, it's a victory amid all the defeats. An important one too.

When your hair falls out during chemotherapy it is a scary, troubling moment; it's brutal, and uncontrolled and happens without warning. Whole handfuls tumble out on clothes, or knot themselves round a hairbrush, or just sit there in twisted clumps on the pillow when you get up in the morning. The violence, the suddenness, is chilling. You think of old photos when it happens, of black-and-white footage of people having their heads shaved, images of oppression, of bullying, fear, loss; a person's identity torn away in fistfuls of hair.

It happened to Vikki when we were on holiday in Scotland on the beautiful island of Mull, several weeks before the support-group meeting. Over dinner one night we found ourselves in discussion with the people sitting nearby. After the normal pleasantries had been exchanged we'd got to talking, where you were from, what you do, and it was established that Vikki was involved in the high-street fashion industry. We quickly moved on to talk about things more widely – though not her cancer – and the evening blossomed. We seemed to have a rapport with that particular couple, which led to a whole evening of conversation, and there was fun, laughter, plenty of gossip and trivia. There, on a remote Scottish island, far away from the hospitals and the tests and the appointments, it was possible, for once, to be normal again.

We retired to bed feeling happy, the only setback being the discovery of a clump of Vikki's hair on her clothes. But we weren't too alarmed. Hair loss might start without warning but its progress is uneven and sometimes takes a while – days, weeks even. Besides, we were having our wig made already, our proper handmade theatrical wig, which would look good, would make her feel strong and confident. We'd be okay.

Our conversation returned to the heart-warming evening spent in beautifully mundane chat with the other couple, and we fell asleep to the sound of the wind that brushed against the windows, blowing away any thoughts of alarm.

By the morning most of Vikki's hair had fallen out. Clumps and clumps of it were now just lying on the pillow in deathly piles. She had great bald patches all over her head and was scared and vulnerable. Mixed with the shock, the sheer open-mouthed this-shouldn't-be-happening terror, was a practical question: how do we deal with it? We're miles from home. Unprepared.

What do we do?

Understandably she didn't want to walk out in public looking like she'd just had her hair cut by Edward Scissorhands. She was still adjusting to the shock of it. But we had nothing to cover it up. No hats, no caps, not even a hoodie. I rooted around, trying to find something, anything that would help as she sat silently on the bed, touching her head, staring at the remains of her old self on the pillow.

Twenty minutes later we appeared in a packed dining room for breakfast. 'Morning,' said our new friends from the previous night. They looked up and froze.

'Morning,' said Vikki, as brazenly as she could muster.

And as we walked through and took our seats, I was aware of the squeak of chairs at other tables as guests turned to look at the newest arrivals.

A man and his wife, who was apparently a big wheel in high-street fashion but whose head was now swathed inexplicably in two bright, clashing tartan scarves, bought as a joke the day before from a tourist shop in Tobermory.

At the support group, Mary claps her hands and the room falls silent. She welcomes everyone, then name-checks a woman with ginger hair sitting three rows back with another, much older, woman holding her hand tightly. The woman with the ginger hair is hunched and taut, just as Vikki was at first, bent over as if sheltering from something – which she is: the terrible news that she has only recently been diagnosed with cancer. She nestles into her chair and people smile kindly at her, then turn back to hear the speaker, whom Mary introduces, a much taller thin woman who looks as if she definitely has her own hair and eyebrows. She is probably forty but is dressed like a sixty-year-old.

'This is Annette,' says Mary. 'She's going to talk about cancer and nutrition.'

Mary sits down and Annette gets to her feet. 'Cancer and nutrition,' she announces. Her voice is dry and passionless, neither harsh nor overly sympathetic. It sounds like a voice that spends a lot of time locked away in labs poring over a microscope. Not a voice that spends a lot of time with other voices.

The first image is flashed up on the screen. It's a picture of a bit of coast with a pipe outlet that is spewing sewage onto a beach. Litter lies at the entrance to the pipe. There is a diseased and dead fish in the foreground, bloated and colourful, its largest eye (one is swollen grotesquely more than the other) bulging and bloodshot. An overweight tourist sits on a deckchair only feet away, seemingly oblivious.

'We live in a world that is terribly polluted,' declares Annette. 'The whole food chain is polluted. Everything we eat is polluted. Everything we drink is polluted.'

There is movement in the seats as people take this in.

Annette then goes into comprehensive detail, outlining how every portion, every morsel, every last drop of the stuff we put into our bodies has been exposed to hormones, toxins, chemicals, agricultural poisons and industrial solvents. And it's not just the food and drink. It's the packaging too – the plastic packaging, the melting, leaking, carcinogenic plastic packaging, the plastic knives and forks, the plastic sandwich boxes, the cling film and the foil that we use to cover food, the plastic bags we carry it all in.

Everything.

There is a moment about twenty minutes into her lecture when there is a change in the atmosphere around the room. At the beginning there was a silence, a reverence, but now there is defiance, a kind of Blitz spirit. There are nudges, knowing winks, pointing fingers and black humour. I see a woman playfully elbow the one next to her, as if to say, 'That's you done for!' In the space of a few minutes the conference room has turned into a 1940s tube station during an air raid.

Finally we get on to hot drinks.

'What about tea?' says a woman, forlornly clutching a huge cup that she has refilled at least twice since she arrived.

'There's nothing wrong with a couple of cups of tea . . .'

'Thank God,' says the woman in the audience. 'I drink loads of it.'

There is a relieved chuckle from the rest of the people around her.

'. . . once or twice a month.' Annette finishes her sentence, and there is an audible gasp from all around. Some murmurs of discontent too.

'But decaffeinated tea is surely all right?' says a posher woman, who sounds as if she decaffeinates her own.

'It depends on how it has been decaffeinated,' replies Annette, doubtfully.

I look around. The recently diagnosed woman with the ginger hair starts to cry. Her friend squeezes her hand harder.

Mary looks concerned.

The general murmurs of discontent grow louder. A large woman in the audience gets to her feet and shuffles to the door.

'If I can just interrupt,' says Mary, getting to her feet, 'I think a number of people here are maybe concerned that you're being a little negative.'

'I'm not trying to be,' says Annette, nonplussed.

'I've just been diagnosed,' says the ginger-haired woman, through her tears. 'I came here because I thought I'd get some support but now . . .' Her voice breaks and she starts to sob loudly.

Half a row of women stand up and head for the exit.

'I think Annette is just saying that we have to be a little careful,' says Mary to the ginger-haired woman, trying to calm things. 'Aren't you, Annette?'

She looks at Annette, her eyes pleading with her to step in and say something.

'I'm just trying to give the facts,' says Annette.

'I think this is just so wrong,' says the ginger-haired woman.

More people get to their feet and shuffle out. Annette watches them go. For the first time something seems to register in her eyes. 'Maybe I'll just leave it there for tonight,' she says.

'Well, er, thank you very much, Annette. Lots of interesting points,' says Mary, hurriedly leading the audience in a desultory round of applause. 'If any of you want to continue talking to Annette I'm sure she'll happily answer questions.'

But no one wants to talk to Annette. No one wants to go anywhere near Annette.

Annette looks a bit confused.

'Next meeting's on Thursday. Same time,' Mary shouts hopefully. 'We've got a talk on support bras.'

The room is nearly empty. Mary makes an attempt to offer a cheery smile and small-talk to people on their way out, as if this is just another evening, but her eyes, which flash angrily a couple of times in Annette's direction, tell another story.

Afterwards, Vikki and I sit in the car, reflecting on the evening. Seeing that newly diagnosed woman so traumatised, so fragile, took us back to the beginning. To that Tuesday morning at Greenwich Hospital when a simple scan turned into something much worse. We start talking about other things too, about our day and how ironic it was that we raced to this meeting only to be fed the gloomy message that we're all doomed because of the food we consume. And then we remember the ready-meal we bolted to enable us to be on time. We think about how the plastic tops didn't come off the containers properly but presumably just melted into the lasagne when we put it into the oven, and how the container had got stuck and we'd had to prise it out. And we think of Annette who is worried about tea that has been decaffeinated in the wrong way.

We start to giggle, hysterically, because we've just eaten a meal of boiled plastic with a hint of lasagne, a horrible unhealthy glutinous mess, a ready-meal of cancer cells. Soon tears of laughter are rolling down our faces, our stomach muscles hurt and our voices are reduced to whispers that erupt into screams as, for those few minutes, we're released from the dark dismal place we now inhabit.

And we're flying again.

14

THE KINDNESS OF STRANGERS

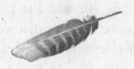

Bereavement fatigue has set in.

I desperately feel the need for a change of scene. To see different people. Have different thoughts. Feel different emotions. There is little I can see or do or touch or think that doesn't lead me back to what has happened. From my upstairs window I can even see the spire of the church marking the cemetery where Vikki is buried.

And now, five months on from her death, I'm screaming inside, crying out for a little inspiration. I'm weary and bored of the dark stuff. The reflection and regret. The 'what-ifs' that come to you at two in the morning. The letters, the cards that still turn up, the heartrending conversations I still have. I'm all burned out.

If there is respite it's tiny, a few hours here, a few hours there. A few hopeful, warm moments in a day before I'm dragged, kicking and screaming, back to the murky pool. I feel dried out. Beaten up. I need something else if only for a few days – a week would be great. Just enough to rest the aching, groaning parts of me that carry the grief around, like a giant boulder.

More importantly I want something else for Romy too. A chance for her to have some fun. A chance to escape. A chance for her and I to have an adventure together. To share the laughter that we've always done in the past. She has seen too much of her serious dad in the last few months, her weighed-down, stressed-out and befuddled dad. She needs the old version back.

I think of a typical Sunday afternoon at home as it used to be, me on all fours climbing up a pile of cushions on the bed, with her on my back urging me on, the two of us screeching with laughter as I tried and failed to get us to the top of that particular mountain. Or transporting her, screaming with excitement on an improvised cart made of an old suitcase around the landing at high speed, or playing Kradar where I had to stop her attacking my kingdom, which was mum and dad's bed, armed only with a pillow. Great fun. Stupid, silly, physical, laugh out loud dad fun. It's something we used to enjoy. It was part of our closeness. But that's all taken a back seat for the time being with all this talk of funerals and arrangements and grieving.

We need a break.

With immaculate timing, my actor friend Gordon Kennedy invites Romy and me out to where he's filming, in Budapest. He's playing Little John in the BBC's production of *Robin Hood*. He suggests we come for a week and stay with him in his flat. This seems an excellent opportunity – we'll be well looked after and entertained with visits to the set and the studios, plus our accommodation is taken care of. It's just what's needed and we're delighted to accept.

It's interesting the way friends react to illness and death. Some run straight towards the fire, offering support and help. Solid, reliable. Exactly as you would expect them to be. Others, surprisingly, move in the opposite direction, perhaps spooked and fearful of what is going on and seeing their own fragility in your situation. Maybe, crushed by what they see as the expectation placed on them, they wait for others to step in. Sometimes they disappear altogether. It isn't predictable as to who falls into which camp. Relative strangers become rocks in the course of long-term illness and bereavement but lifelong friends can disappear, never to be seen or heard of again.

I used to assume that everyone would pull together in a time of crisis. After all, that's what you do, isn't it? Apparently not. I was surprised at an early support group meeting that Vikki and I attended to be told of the very high rate of divorce or separation among couples, one of whom has recently been diagnosed. Mortality or the threat of it does weird things to the human psyche.

My experience of friends proves, happily, completely positive. I'm fortunate in encountering no surprises at all. No friends backing away or hiding. No reservations (save for the man who couldn't get over it and his reluctance remains a source of comedy rather than upset). In fact it's quite the opposite. We've been showered with love and support since the moment of Vikki's death – from all directions.

I think of Vikki's sister, Patricia, whose unfailing attention and practical support keeps us going through many dark times. Her help is given selflessly, without question or demand. She asks nothing for herself. There is no charge. No angle. There is just her love for her sister, her care and concern for me and her amazing devotion to her niece.

I think, too, of Romy's godmother, Morwenna, always sensitive and a wonderful listener. She is considerate, utterly dependable and a true friend to me too. A wise counsel. A star.

And there are dozens of others who make their contributions: a thoughtful headmistress, sensitive teachers, the redoubtable PTA, kind neighbours, friends we barely knew before who step up magnificently. We find ourselves borne up by a wave of love and support, and our small Norfolk world gathers round us and envelops us in its old-fashioned sense of community, its 1950s sense of the simplicity of the world.

People in need. Must help.

Without cynicism. Without complication.

People in need. Must help.

And now there is Gordon too, just the person you want to be your guide on your first trip alone out of the country – relentlessly optimistic, energetic, full of life.

In Budapest he is – typically – one of the central figures on the production, despite having nowhere near the biggest part. He is known to everyone, as friendly with the Hungarian stuntmen who speak little English as he is with the Sheriff of Nottingham. Nothing is too much trouble for Gordon. Everything is within reach. It's like being away with a kindly uncle. And from the moment we arrive till the moment we leave, the whole trip is an exercise in regeneration.

Everywhere we go on the production we are welcomed with warmth and sensitivity. At the Hungarian film studios Romy is whisked away by Maid Marian and spends hours watching her having her makeup done – every young girl's dream. Then we are driven up into the Hungarian mountains with the cast, through the lush trees, dense woodland and leafy valleys, and watch as horsemen gallop through the fog, yelling and brandishing swords. All of the actors write sweet messages in the scrapbook that Romy carries. They draw little cartoons too and pose for pictures. Then as they wait for their call for the next scene, they join Romy and me in a spot of den building. Later, we're invited out for dinner with Gordon, by Maid Marian and her family, who are also visiting and there we are fêted and embraced and made to feel like guests of honour. At the end of the night Romy is presented with gifts – a beautiful handmade Hungarian folk tiara and an exquisite embroidered silk doll.

On other days Romy and I spend time together, just the two of us, exploring the city, walking down the wide boulevards, visiting the old Communist square, with its massive statues, then the Palace of Wonders where she solves giant maths puzzles and bounces on an enormous mat supported by bungee ropes. We go to a renowned confectioner, stuff gorgeous truffles into our mouths and I take pictures of Romy laughing, her face smothered in chocolate. Then we're dipping into the sharp turquoise blue of an open-air swimming pool and she squeals with delight, thundering down spectacular water slides and disappearing into the soft surf to emerge with her arms raised in triumph.

It is the most effortless of holidays, and as we're driven back to the airport I feel encouraged and relieved. Just for a few days I've been away from home. Away from the pressures of being a widower. I've taken back some life, the kind of life I'd forgotten it was possible to have, one of laughter, adventure and people other than nurses, doctors, funeral directors, vicars and solicitors.

I've eaten out in restaurants, seen new sights, enjoyed happy times with my daughter again, felt part of a different narrative away from the bereavement story, the years of illness, the hospitals, the unending grinding process of deterioration and death. You never completely forget your grief and even though I'm away it's still there, like a rude uninvited guest who refuses to leave – at night, during the day, even when I'm talking to other people. But I've had glimpses of something else, too, just for a few days. And for that I'm incredibly grateful.

We get home and enjoy the TV series when it comes out. Later when there's a storyline in which Maid Marian dies, the actress who plays the part writes a beautiful letter in advance of its broadcast, addressed to Romy, concerned that she'll be upset. She reassures Romy that it's only a story, emphasising that it's the character who dies not her. She hopes that Romy won't be too distraught and sends her love. It's the latest in a series of well-judged, sensitive gestures that we'll always associate with that trip and those people.

The kindness of strangers.

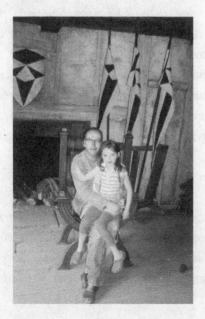

15

THE SCAN

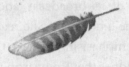

It always starts like this, with the sick feeling two weeks before the appointment. It feels as if an invisible hand is pulling my stomach muscles tight, squeezing them into a ball. As the days pass and the date looms, the squeezing is more persistent, and the hand seems to reach upwards as well, stretching its fingers to draw in my shoulder blades, my back, my heart and my ribs, pulling and squeezing harder and harder till I'm a tight, locked mass of twisted fibres and mashed-up bone. My breathing shortens and the nausea ebbs and flows.

We're here for the yearly scan.

Much has happened in the six years since the original diagnosis in Greenwich, since the operation and the chemotherapy. Vikki has had six-monthly checks, which have gone well, and yearly scans, which have been clear. Her hair has grown back, though it is now wiry and curly whereas before it had been smooth and straight. She thinks it feels like someone else's. Possibly Fatima Whitbread's.

But she is cancer-free. At the moment she is cancer-free. And that is all that matters.

Her prognosis is good. The original cancer was dealt with. The scans on the other parts of her body were clear as well. She now has every prospect of good health and a long life. So, we have left hospitals behind and started anew. Moving on. Rebuilding. Renewing. We have tried to forget the traumas and shocks, tried to recover our optimism and ambition. And over this six-year period I know we have succeeded.

We've bought ourselves a bolthole on the north Norfolk coast and acquired a new, invigorating country life. Vikki has taken a career break and we've spent more time together. We've travelled, we've seen in the Millennium, we've partied, danced and laughed.

And, best of all, most incredibly, most magically, we've done what we've both wanted to do for a long time: we've become parents.

Our daughter, Romy, is christened on a stunning September Sunday in St Alfege's Church in Greenwich, with the sun streaming through the windows, bathing the onlookers in glorious sunlight. Romy is a true miracle baby. Vikki was told many times that she was highly unlikely to conceive having been through chemotherapy, and when she got pregnant and gave birth, it felt as if something in the universe had been rebalanced, something repaid in our favour.

Romy wears a long white satin gown and delicate little white scratch mittens that make her look like a child from a Victorian novel. We stand proudly in the middle of the aisle, Vikki holding her, me leaning in, lost in helpless adoration, while her godparents flank her on both sides in a loose semi-circle. As the vicar speaks her name and dabs her forehead gently with water, Romy doesn't gurgle or cry out, she smiles just like her mum; inscrutable and self-contained.

Afterwards, we leave the church and walk up the hill to the small hotel that nestles among the fine Georgian houses that circle Blackheath. There, in a large panelled dining room, we sit, eat and chat, close family mingling with old friends, a sumptuous, joyful atmosphere pervading the room, crackling with laughter and enthusiasm, the conversation full of zip and energy; a new life celebrated, a new hope, the outlook as bright as the warm sunshine that continues to peer in through the large, elegant windows.

At the end of the afternoon everyone gathers for one last celebratory moment as I stand at the front of the assembled party holding Romy, with Vikki alongside me, and invite people to raise a glass. As I speak, I find myself scanning the crowd, taking in all the smiling, approving faces, wanting to record the moment for ever. I finish my sweep of the room and notice Vikki at my shoulder. She isn't looking at me, she is utterly transfixed by the little girl in my arms, smiling at her with an expression of wonderment and disbelief. I can feel the warmth of my daughter's body against my side and the warmth of Vikki's gaze, and for a few gorgeous seconds I feel the strength of our bond, the three of us so close we're almost a single being, bound together with love.

It's a perfect moment.

Now, it's three years after the christening; it's summer and we're back for our latest yearly scan. And that bliss, that contentment, is on hold for we're still vulnerable, still fearful. No matter that we're some distance now from the original diagnosis, with a bunch of successful scans behind us. Our new, bright, optimistic life suddenly feels threatened. It always does at this time of year. We will probably always feel like this. Even in ten or twenty years. Even when we're into middle age, and other illnesses, other dangers, start to beckon.

There is no absolute certainty with cancer, no ultimate cure. At least, not now. Maybe one day. The cancer could come back. Just because Vikki has been well doesn't mean she always will be. The uncertainty eats away at us again as we approach the latest appointment.

In the days before, life seems to slow down and stop. It's difficult to focus on anything other than the scan. You can't contemplate anything beyond it. Events in the diary booked in after that date seem somehow unreal. As if they're floating somewhere in the future. Ethereal and slight in the face of the hulking concrete barrier we now have to get beyond.

It's suddenly all about the scan. Just that twenty minutes.

Twenty minutes in every year that defines the year and all the years after. Twenty minutes that can propel us forward or drag us back to a dark place of uncertainty and worry.

'Are you going away this year?' says the radiographer, as he runs the probe over Vikki's breast.

We're in a small room at the hospital. She's lying on the bed. He is to her left side peering at a screen as he scans her. I'm on the other side of the bed, holding her hand and trying not to look at the screen.

He scans each breast in turn, squeezing the gel from a tube onto her skin then running the probe over it. He has already scanned one breast so we're halfway through.

'Yes,' she answers.

'Whereabouts?'

'Sicily.'

Mark, the radiographer, is a genial curly-haired guy of about fifty. I like to hear his everyday conversation as he does the scan. It makes it all feel normal. As if nothing is wrong. But I hate it if he pauses or doesn't answer a question straight away. Then I start to panic. Some radiographers will talk all the way through in a bid to keep the patient calm, but from the beginning we've agreed with Mark that he'll tell us straight away if there's a problem.

The probe moves towards a different part of her breast. 'I've – er . . . ' Mark zips it back to where it was previously.

I look up anxiously at the screen. He's going back on something. Why?

He looks hard at the screen and cocks his head at an

*angle, as if assessing something. He takes the probe off Vikki
altogether, then puts it down again in the same spot.*

Please, God, no.

*'. . . never been to Sicily,' he continues, moving the probe
to another part of the breast.*

He's moved on. He's speaking. We're okay.

She grips my hand hard. I grip it harder in return.

*'I've done the northern bit of Italy, the lakes. That was
nice – Lake Como.'*

He must be nearly done. Surely.

He moves around. Black blobs appear on the screen.

I catch sight of them. My heart almost stops.

'Cysts,' he says. Then he moves off again.

*'I'm not really an Italy person, more a Spain one,' he
continues.*

*We've been going for nearly ten minutes. Feels like an
hour. Surely he must be nearly finished. Surely.*

*'Done Madrid, Barcelona,' he continues. 'Never Valencia.
Okay . . .'*

*It's an 'okay' that sounds relaxed. An 'okay' that speaks
of conclusion, satisfaction. Finishing. The pilot has brought
the plane safely into land.*

*Vikki lets go of my hand. I see that my palm is white
and there are red marks where she has been pressing.*

'Okay,' he says again.

*This second 'okay' sounds even more conclusive than the
last.*

'If we just . . . er . . .' He moves the probe an inch to the

right and wiggles in his seat as if he's preparing a bigger move – to get up. To pack up and leave.

I can feel my heart start to accelerate. I can feel the anticipation of what is to come – I can feel it on the very edge of my lips. Sweet like wine.

He's going to remove the probe. Remove the probe, wipe the end, then offer Vikki a kitchen roll. She'll tear a piece off and wipe herself. A bit indelicate but we never care by that point because that means it's over and the relief is huge. Then he will talk about forwarding the results to her oncologist just as a matter of record, as a way of comparing for future scans, but we won't hear that: we'll be thinking only of getting outside and hugging, kissing, celebrating and every bit of life we now have permission to live.

'Erm . . .'

But the probe has stopped again. Still on her.

'Hang on,' he says.

God. No. Please.

Please move the probe off. Tell us it's a cyst. Mark shuffles forward a little on his seat and peers closer at the screen. There is a silence that probably lasts ten seconds but feels like half an hour.

She grabs my hand again. I feel my heart sinking down to my boots. 'I don't like the look of that,' *he says.*

A moment, a tiny moment among talk of holidays and thoughts of hope, fun and renewal, a moment that erupts with a crack, like a starting pistol, setting you off down a different path.

'No, I don't like that at all.'

Vikki's face has frozen and I am paralysed too, because we know what that means. Instinctively. We don't need the actual words.

Mark looks at us. 'I'm sorry,' he says. 'I'm really sorry.'

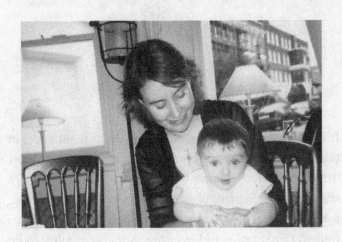

THE OWL AT THE WINDOW

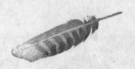

It is a winter's day six months after the funeral and I'm taking my daughter to school. We have argued and now there is an icy silence between us. The wrath of a six-year-old is like that of an eighty-year-old. Remorseless, forensic, fierce. And now she sits on the stairs, arms folded, cross, as I stand over her. She has a point, to be fair.

Sometimes, unfortunately, I'm not gentle enough when I'm doing her hair, and when a tangle gets caught in the brush, I pull it too hard in a bid to get rid of the knot, rather than gently tugging at it with small, shallow strokes. She has told me before, many times, but I have forgotten again in the rush and she has rightly reprimanded me.

But I'm tired as well. Tired as it is possible to be only when you're grieving. When your limbs ache and you're tired in your dreams and you wake not with a crisp, clear head but a throb in your bones and mud in your veins.

I'm tired too because it's just me now. Just me. A lone parent with a six-year-old. No one else to sew the label on, book the dance lesson, clear up the sick, cajole, understand, sympathise, be stern. There's just me. Depleted, ruffled and edgy. So I forgot the hair instruction and caught a tangle, and she has howled the place down and folded her arms and refused to allow her hair to be done any more. We're caught in an ugly stalemate. Me, standing helplessly over her with the brush in hand. She, with arms folded in defiant refusal. And I can feel the tension rise up my spine to my neck, grabbing the back of my head in angry white knuckles. I am trapped, stuck. And my heart goes out to her too, frustrated and cross, her hair pulled about painfully yet again by a cack-handed amateur. All she wants is the silken touch of her mum. All she gets is the clumsiness of her dad.

How do we get out of this?

There's no sharpness, no brightness in my head. I see no solutions, just a problem, and I feel myself sinking, the weight on my back pulling me down.

'Don't worry about the hair,' I say. I unlock the door and let her out. A rush of cold air hits me. A cold, clean blast from across the wide field next to my house. You can see the trees sway in the distance, hear the soft hiss of the wind as it weaves through the conifers. I reach in my back pocket for my keys. The car is where I left it last night at an angle to the house near to the front door. 'In you get' I say.

I click the car door open and quickly turn back to the house to lock the door. As I do so, I realise my daughter has barely moved but is standing several feet away from the car, looking at it. I follow her gaze and see why she has stopped. *All the windows are wound down. All of them. Right down to the bottom.* On this cold, clear day. I never open the windows, even in the height of summer – it's a standing joke among my friends – and I certainly wouldn't ever think of opening them in winter. I'm puzzled. I know I left the car last night with all the windows shut. How could this have happened?

'Probably something wrong with the electrics,' I say. Inside, though, I am not convinced.

I take her to school and we talk about other things but my mind is still on the windows. How could it happen? How? Actually, physically, practically, *how*?

On the way back, I search out every possibility. Could I have been responsible for the windows? Is it possible I just decided to air the car? But I would never, ever do that. And it's impossible to do it by accident. There is no single button that controls all the windows. You would have to depress four, have four 'accidents'. Could it have been a malfunction? Possibly. But everything seems to be working fine again – I shut all the windows and test all the buttons. Nothing wrong. Could it have been a freak electric storm? Absolutely not: it was a calm, placid night.

Now, I'm no mystic. When odd things like this happen my mind does not automatically think of spirits or unseen forces. If there is an inexplicable event I generally look for rational explanations and find them. Or if I can't I'm normally just happy to let them be.

And yet . . .

On this particular cold winter morning I get the strangest feeling – a kind of glow, a warmth that fills me from my head to my feet, a calm that descends like a blanket, covering me, holding me, enveloping me. I'm not imagining it. I can feel the warmth as readily as if I were standing next to a fire. And along with this sensation comes the total conviction – clear, unblinking, realised not just as a passing thought but as an instinctive certainty, like the firmness of a road beneath your feet or the sharp pain of a paper cut – that Vikki is involved in this somehow. Playful, mischievous and reassuring.

I feel this so strongly at this specific moment in time, with no scientific evidence at all, that if you held a gun to my head I'd swear blind that there's no other possible explanation for it. It's Vikki. It just has to be. She's close and she's reaching out to me, cajoling me, reassuring me, lifting the gloom. Telling me she's there. Urging me not to worry. Making it all feel better.

I feel it. I know it.

I'm overwhelmed by a sense of well-being, the ache in my back has gone, as has the feeling of being trapped. I am lifted. I am inspired. I feel good.

The whole day takes on a brighter aspect. I feel purposeful. I feel I can move forward. I even feel I can cope with the knots in my lovely daughter's hair.

I am restored.

Hysteria? Maybe. The madness of grief? Possibly. But every time I recall that day I can experience it again – return in a second to the same warmth running through my veins, the same strange calm, and the same over-whelming sense of her *there*.

Just *there*.

A few weeks later, I'm woken at first light by a sound from the landing outside my bedroom. Where I live, out in the country, surrounded by fields and woods, I'm used to certain noises – the cry of a deer, the rustling of the trees, the crack of the wooden floorboards in my house contracting in the cold – but this is something quite different.

It starts as a scratching sound but then there is rustling and a thump. There is a short pause, then all three sounds return but they seem more urgent, the scratching more intense, the rustling more feverish, the thumping more forceful. I'm immediately puzzled. My daughter is staying with a friend so I'm alone in the house. And it isn't the sound of a rodent in the attic or another person outside – here, in the eccentric countryside, I have a window-cleaner who turns up unannounced and just appears at the window with his squeegee. No, it's definitely something different. Something insistent. Something energetic and urgent. And something big.

I get up, put on a dressing-gown and go out of the bedroom door, bleary-eyed and a little apprehensive. Outside, the landing wraps around a central staircase that leads downstairs. It forms a carpeted square, round which you can walk. On either side of the landing, shelves are stuffed with children's books, old files, photo albums, school art projects and stacks of magazines. At the far end, opposite, a sofa faces my bedroom. Above it, there is a large landscape-shaped window, looking out on to the front garden and the row of Leylandii that runs along its edge. My gaze is immediately drawn to it.

But, then, it couldn't fail to be.

The bird has a wing span of three or four feet, and is hovering majestically outside the house, big enough to fill the three large panes of glass that make up the window. Its body is white and its wings are topped with brown feathers. Its beak is curved and black and looks razor sharp, as do its claws, which seem disproportionately large. Its eyes are huge, unblinking and dark. But the most extraordinary thing is its face, which is heart-shaped.

Every few seconds it moves forward, wings flapping towards the glass. Then its body makes contact and literally bounces off, returning to its original position. A barn owl is trying to get into my house.

I've seen barn owls around – they're common in this part of Norfolk – and I've heard them many times, but I've never encountered one in daylight. And I've never come across one trying to get into my house. As I watch, it seems to increase its efforts, retreating a few feet further away, then flying into the glass with an even louder thump. After the second of these collisions, it arches its spine, so its head is tilted back, its belly is pointed at the window and its legs are further forward. It scratches furiously at the glass, its legs pumping like pistons. Then it repeats the whole cycle, retreating, slamming into the glass and scratching. It really, really wants to get in now.

I haven't moved since I first appeared on the landing. I've remained frozen in the doorway of my bedroom, watching, fascinated, a little apprehensive but much more thrilled. Now I want to take a closer look. I feel I *must* get closer. I edge forward towards the window, but as soon as I do, the owl seems to notice and lessens its ferocious scrabbling.

I take one further step forward and it quietens – its wings seem slower, its headlong rush into the glass more of a glide, as if it's automatic, a reflex action, less important now. I take another two tentative steps forward. I don't want to alarm the owl and frighten it away. Quite the opposite. I want it to stay. As I draw nearer, the owl seems to stop its frantic motion. Now it is content to hover.

For a few odd seconds (I have no idea how long), we face each other in a strange suspended moment that is tranquil yet simmering with energy, me motionless, halfway towards the window but shivering with excitement, the bird hovering, wings flapping; still, yet powerful too. No longer the frustrated, scratching, flapping creature it was at the beginning but regal and assured, as if it could smash through the glass at will but has decided not to.

Suddenly, without warning, the owl retreats, turns and, with an energetic crescendo of its wings, sweeps off. I run to the window just in time to see that graceful, elegant creature disappear into the dark woods on the other side of the road at the front of the house. The sky looks very empty.

I'm wide awake now and, as I slump down on the sofa, the sun's rays are pushing sharply and brightly through the twisted fingers of the Leylandii. They pour through the window above my head throwing a spotlight back across the landing to where I have been standing, bathing the scene with a golden glow.

Then as I sit and contemplate the strange event a familiar warm feeling starts to course through me again and I feel that sense of having witnessed something powerful and irresistible that involves Vikki. I don't understand it but I

Carl Gorham

don't have to. I feel its truth. She is near again, and I am with her, and our worlds are connected, and for a few seconds we are close again. Within a breath.

17

FASTER AND FASTER

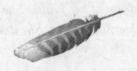

We're in Hong Kong and it's 2007, three years on from the scan that dragged us back to the cancer world, the afternoon that had started so promisingly, with talk of holidays in Sicily and Spain, then turned so cruelly sour. We're in a different race now. A very different race.

Since the cancer reappeared Vikki has had further chemotherapy but the cancer just wouldn't leave her alone. A year after it reappeared for the first time, it was back again and she had to have yet more treatment – a mastectomy and some radiotherapy. When she was discharged from hospital in 2005, the medical data we had accumulated was telling us that although she was cancer-free at that moment, there was a greatly increased chance of it returning in the future.

What was more, we knew that if it came back again it wouldn't go away.

It was just too persistent. Too virulent. Too angry.

So she agreed a special programme of monitoring with her consultant, a programme that suited her and the person she was – positive, determined and realistic. She agreed to go and see him every few months for a general examination and detailed discussion of her health. She didn't obsessively scan. She didn't obsessively check. She didn't go looking for the cancer.

Why would she?

She didn't want to know if it came back because there was nothing she could do about it if it did and she didn't want to spend whatever time was left worrying about the end. In any case, there was no absolute guarantee that the cancer would return, though it was highly likely. She might survive well into the future – we just didn't know. If that proved correct, she also didn't want to waste those years going in and out of hospitals.

Besides, she was sick of cancer, of hospitals and consultants, of constant testing and results. The build-up, the anticipation, the terror, the explosions of adrenaline, the relief, the whole, ugly, sickening juggernaut. The way it dominated her life. She just wanted to get away. She just wanted to start living again.

So she took the brave decision, the only one she could, being the person she was, to get back some element of control – to battle it on her terms. She made regular visits to the consultant, swallowed a new and powerful drug every day in pill form, which we hoped would stave off the cancer's return, and we gritted our teeth and crossed our fingers whenever she got a cough or a pain, lest it be something more sinister.

And 'She's well.' That was what we could say. 'She's well at the moment.'

That was all we could say.

So, we're in a different race now. We're running, running, trying to stay ahead of it. And time feels different. It seems to race by. Days. Weeks. Months. Faster and faster. We have no time to lose. Because life is uncertain. We don't wait. We do. We travel. We party. We explore. We live.

We go to a TV awards ceremony and both get so drunk that I fall into a table and Vikki falls in the snow outside. We take our daughter to football matches and teach her to shout at the ref. We move house again and settle in Norfolk full time, leaving London behind. We try canoeing, go ballooning, build bonfires on the beach, ski and ice skate.

We join the PTA at school, raise money for charity, make new friendships. We hold parties, take hundreds of photos and celebrate every moment that races by as we try to catch time and hold it. We live our lives more intensely, more hectically, more fully than ever before. We don't look over our shoulders.

Last year we visited Palm Springs, San Francisco, Las Vegas. Now we're in Hong Kong. Soon we'll move on to Australia. A once-in-a-lifetime trip. Let's do it now. No time to lose.

We go to the top of the Peninsula Hotel and look out over

Hong Kong harbour – shimmering lights, energy, life. We go shopping and on boat trips. We go to Kowloon Park. All around us there is colour, noise and bustle. But Vikki can't seem to shake the jetlag. I'm okay and so is Romy, but Vikki isn't over it at all.

Next it's Australia and we get to Sydney and to the Opera House, a vast jaw-dropping wooden beehive. There we see 'The Marriage of Figaro', an amazing spectacle. We go to the zoo to meet the ten most poisonous snakes in the world, to Manly beach where picture-perfect blonde surfers battle the waves. We go to a fair at the waterside where one of the rides shoots out over Sydney Harbour, then back again. But still Vikki can't get over the jetlag.

On and on we go. Faster and faster.

We travel on to Adelaide where Romy and I make shadow puppets on the walls of our rented cottage while Vikki rests, and then we visit the beautiful Cricket Ground where Romy gets to operate the scoreboard – and all I'm thinking when I gaze at my tired-looking wife is, Please be over it. Please. But still . . .

We go to a wildlife park and a kangaroo tries to steal the bag I'm carrying. For a second I'm in an absurd tug of war match with Australia's national symbol while everyone around laughs and takes pictures.

Fun. Laughter. Fear. Worry.

Faster and faster.

We travel into the Barossa Valley, where we celebrate Romy's birthday with Disney costumes galore. There are wine-tastings, walks and epic drives through huge valleys, with vast mountains on either side. Then we head along the coast through long stretches of uninhabited wasteland, where we travel for hours with barely a human sighting, just the forlorn roadkill at the side of the highway.

Maybe it's not jetlag. Maybe it's something else.

We head to Melbourne on the final leg of our journey, Vikki now too weak to share any of the driving. At times she can bearly read the map. The narrow coastal road becomes wider. More cars join, and there are two, three, up to six lanes. More and more vehicles, vans now and lorries too. Huge pantechnicons appear on either side, and our small rented car feels as if it's drowning amongst the giants. Several times we have to take evasive action.

It's the worst of drives, like a drive into Hell.

In Melbourne, Vikki doesn't leave the hotel room. We get a doctor, who talks vaguely about a virus. Neither of us believes him.

Faster and faster.

On to the last night in Melbourne, the last one before our flight home, and things seem to slow down. Just for a few hours. After the stress of the previous few days, after the fears, the constant glances in Vikki's direction, a beautifully ordinary evening takes place, emerging out of the fog, exceptional by its very mundanity, the two of us watching Aussie Rules football on TV while Romy sleeps soundly next door.

It's as if we're back at the beginning. As if the intervening *years have changed nothing, leaving just the two of us, sparking, joking, sharing the moment, enjoying each other's company; as if we're back in the college room at Oxford, eating cheese-and-coleslaw jacket potato and supping home brew.*

We find ourselves sharing truths and fears, apologising for bad temper and past anger. We're open with each other, and we talk about It, the cancer. We haven't talked about it for a while. We've each thought about it a lot but we've not discussed it openly. Too frightened probably and sick of the subject.

We know that when we get home there will be scans and possibly bad news but for now we still have each other and a sense that we belong at that moment in that space and time. We're grateful for that.

I will always be grateful for that.

Finally the night draws in, the game on the TV ends and Vikki starts to get drowsy. I help her into bed and sit with her as the light fades and the sky goes black. Soon she is fast asleep. Then I check the bags that are already packed and count the passports on the coffee table.

And I feel quite alone.

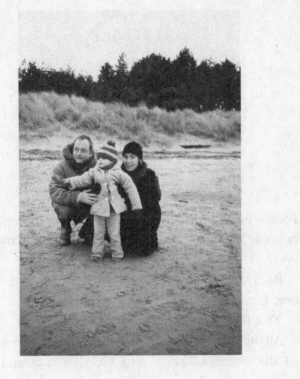

18

STRESSED

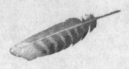

I feel a pain in my chest: my heart rattling my ribcage. I crumple and lie on the floor in the hall. Is it my turn now?

Romy runs into the living room holding her hands over her ears in terror.

This is it. It must be.

All the years of shock – the years of Vikki's treatment, all the moments when your blood freezes and your chest explodes. Years of it. Years and years. All coming back at this one moment. All that stress, of watching, helpless, someone else's suffering. Helpless but still trying to help, wanting to help. The diagnosis, the operations, the chemotherapy, the radiotherapy that followed the check-ups, the X-rays, the scans; the fear, the anticipation, the relief, then the gradual, growing, gnawing fear again. Is it worse? Is it better? Is it there? Is it gone? Is it back? The creeping tentacles of cancer.

All of that shock has been rolled up into one giant ball and is steaming into me now, smashing at my ribcage till it feels as if it's caving in, making my heart pound, my nerves tight, my muscles scream.

I'm on the phone to the ambulance switchboard.

They are ridiculously calm. 'Where is the pain, Mr Gorham?'

'It's in my chest.'

'Do you have pins and needles up your arm?'

'No. But it feels as if there's a ton weight on my chest.'

'We'll have someone with you as soon as possible. Just try not to panic.'

I look through the glass of the hallway door into the living room – Romy still has her hands over her ears but she's looking anxiously at me, tears streaming down her face. I'd give anything for her not to witness this – her only remaining parent lying on the floor of the hallway clutching his chest – but it's too late.

I worry about the effect that these moments of shuddering trauma will have on her. There have been too many moments like this. She is just a little girl; she should be laughing at dogs playing in the park.

'There it goes again!' I can hear the panic in my own voice.

'We'll be with you as soon as possible.'

'Please. Do you know how long?' It must be a heart attack. *Must* be.

'Not long.'

Try not to panic. Breathe.

Romy comes towards the glass and peers through it. I look up into her eyes but she can't bear to see me and runs away again, back down through the living room, out through a door at the far end and up the stairs.

I want to run after her, to take her in my arms, but I have to stay on the floor, curled up in a ball. If I attempt to stand up I'll just blow apart. I need the oak floorboards.

I manage to dial a friend on my mobile, a school mum who lives nearby. She has a spare key. 'It's Carl. I'm not very well.' I try not to sound hysterical but I can't stop the quiver in my voice. 'Can you come? Please? The paramedics are on the way.' I turn over and hold the floor with my arms out, like a starfish.

Minutes pass, I don't know how many. I can only measure time in the waves of chest pain that break over my ribcage. There have been three or four when there is the sound of a key turning in a lock. My friend looks shocked when she sees me lying on the floor. She walks in and kneels down. 'Where does it hurt?'

'My chest,' I say.

She takes my hand while her children hang back at the door, afraid.

I grip it tightly. 'Please find Romy. She's—'

'Just relax,' she says. She looks up. 'Come in,' she says to her children. They don't move. 'Come in!'

For the first time I hear the fear in her voice too.

'Go and find Romy. Quickly now!' she adds.

The children tiptoe past and into the living room, then up the stairs in search of my daughter.

There is a knock at the front door, which is ajar. 'Mr Gorham?'

It's a paramedic.

'Down here,' says my friend.

'Okay, Mr Gorham. What's your first name?'

'It's Carl,' says my friend, gently.

'Okay, Carl, you just stay there.' He kneels and does some quick checks, takes my pulse. 'You've been having chest pains, I understand.'

'Yes, and I can't breathe.'

He looks me over again. 'No pins and needles?'

'No pins and needles.'

'Constant pain? Stabbing pain?'

'There was a stabbing to start with. But it's now more of an ache. Like there's a weight on me.'

'Just in your chest or is it moving around?'

'In my chest.'

The paramedic has a cool, unhurried manner, almost delicate. He checks me over thoroughly. 'Okay, if we can just get you up . . . very slowly.'

I feel calmer already. He wouldn't be moving me if he thought I was dying.

He and my friend help me to my knees, then take an arm each and lead me, shuffling like an old man, into the living room and onto the sofa. I can still feel the tightness in my chest and shoulders. The paramedic gently helps to remove my shirt, then takes out an ECG machine and sticks two wires on my chest.

'Yes, it took me a bit longer to get here than I thought,' he says. 'Especially for a Sunday morning. There's been an accident at Bodham. The A148 is completely clogged up. Doesn't take much, does it?' He watches the ECG go through its paces. 'Reckon I'll have to go back via Gresham. I hope I'm in time for Sunday lunch. It's lamb. My favourite.'

For several minutes there is nothing but the whirring sound of the machine. I glance at my friend who is also looking at it intently. I manage a faint smile.

I look down towards the far end of the room, at the doorway through which the kids disappeared. I can hear some whispers and I can see the edge of a child's leg in the corner of the door frame. A head peaks round and below it, another pair of eyes cautiously appears.

Finally there's a beeping sound and the paramedic tears off a paper printout, then takes the wires off my chest and disconnects the machine. 'The ECG is clear. So, no problems there. To be honest, as soon as I saw you in the hall I didn't think it was a heart problem.'

'Really?' Suddenly I feel like a fraud.

'Yes, you can generally tell.'

'So what do you think happened?' asks my friend.

'A severe panic attack. See a lot of them, these days.

We're all under stress, aren't we? Have you been under stress recently?'

'For about the last ten years,' I say.

He stands, wraps the wires around the ECG machine and packs it away in his holdall. 'Okay. I'll do a report and pass it on to your doctor. You'll need to follow it up with him. Obviously if you have any problems let us know, but for now I'd just say relax as much as possible and take it easy, very easy.'

The children all appear in the doorway.

'You can come in now,' says my friend.

Romy enters cautiously, followed by the other two, her hands no longer over her ears. She walks towards me slowly, kneels down at my side and gently kisses my forehead. I wrap my arms around her and hold her tight. I don't want the hug to ever end.

'I'm going to be all right,' I whisper to her.

'Thank you,' says my friend to the paramedic, as he fastens up his bag.

'No problem. My pleasure.'

As he goes he shoots me a glance. 'What do you do for a living, Mr Gorham?'

'I'm a comedy writer.'

'Really. Anything I'd know?'

'I wrote something called *Stressed Eric*. About the most stressed man in the world.'

He smiles at me. 'Based on you, is it?'

19

HONG KONG

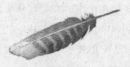

We're running. Running. My daughter and I are running through Hong Kong airport. We're on our way home from Australia and are supposed to be spending a couple of days here again before heading back to England.

But everything is different now.

We haven't even picked up our bags, we've just shouted at a bemused member of the airport staff to get them from the carousel. We need someone else to look after them for we have other much more important things to do.

We have to get in an ambulance.

The doors are open, and Vikki is already inside. Two Chinese paramedics sit at either side of her. The airport staff are standing outside the ambulance waving us frantically on, like runners to the finishing line. We get to the ambulance, climb up the steps and get in. Vikki is lying on a trolley, eyes closed, an oxygen mask strapped tightly to her face. That morning, at breakfast, she was so looking forward to getting here, looking forward to taking her daughter to Hong Kong Disneyland, the final treat of our memorable once-in-a-life-time holiday.

Now she is dying.

The doors slam shut behind us and the ambulance lurches off. No one says where we're going. No one says what's happening. No one says anything. The two paramedics write on clipboards. Take her pulse. Then one mutters something to the other in Chinese and leans forward, holding out his hand towards me. 'Passport?'

I hand over the passports and he takes them without acknowledgement, leafing through all three carefully and making notes on his clipboard. Then he puts his clipboard down. He doesn't give the passports back. Neither does he explain why.

The ambulance rattles on, faster now. Every few seconds there's a bump on the uneven road that makes us all jump out of our seats at the same time, then sit down again. The drip in her arm sways. The Chinese paramedics don't say a word. My heart is racing.

Romy is sitting next to me. I have my arm around her and I keep pulling her in as tight as I can. I'm trying to hold Vikki's hand too but it's awkward because I'm half sitting, half off the seat that runs down one side of the ambulance. I'm desperate not to let go of either of them.

I just mustn't let go.

Then it hits me, an overwhelming sense of blind panic,

the kind that wants to grab hold of something or someone and just collapse into them.

But I can't.

Because it's just me and my daughter and my poor sick wife.

And I've got to keep my head.

Through the narrow window the tower blocks rush by. They're all different sizes but they're all grey and shabby, with washing lines that criss-cross the narrow spaces between them. You can see exactly what's going on inside them: a mother is feeding her child, a family is arguing, pointing, furious, an old man on a balcony is staring blankly down at the street below. All those lives are continuing, absorbed in their dramas, unaware of ours. I want to shout at them.

I want them to help.

We seem to be on a motorway and I feel as if we're heading out of town but there's nothing I can do. The paramedics continue to talk in Chinese and they have our passports. I squeeze my wife's hand. She doesn't respond.

She can't because she's already in a coma.

The nightmare started some nine hours before when Vikki was sick in the car on the way to Melbourne airport, just as we were starting our return journey.

She was sick again as we went through Customs. We wondered if we should wait to see a doctor there but we were desperate to get home and decided to keep going.

If we can just keep going . . .

That was all we were thinking about. Getting home. Being home. The warm comforting arms of home.

But on the plane she got worse. She felt dizzy. She had a pain in her abdomen. She went to the toilet and didn't come out for ages. I had to look for her and help her back to her seat on unsteady legs.

She said she must have fainted. She thought she might have hit her head on the toilet door.

Back in the seat, I tried to make her as comfortable as possible. I massaged her neck. I talked to her. Tried to distract her. I got the steward to bring her extra water. I tried to comfort Romy too. Playing 'I spy'. Trying to sound normal and unworried. Trying not to panic her.

'Is Mummy all right?' asked Romy.

'Mummy's a bit unwell,' I replied.

The hours passed as I held Vikki's hand. Sometimes she slept and sometimes she could talk lucidly to me, but at others she just stared ahead blankly. On a couple of occasions she said odd things that made little sense. At one point she got angry and shouted at me for no reason.

I was bewildered, still trying to be as normal as possible with Romy, watching films with her and drawing on a small pad, then putting my arm around her and gently singing her favourite song as she fell asleep. Inside, though, I was struggling to understand.

Is this a separate unconnected illness? I asked myself.

Is this a symptom of something much worse?

Is this the 'something much worse'?

Should we stay in Hong Kong and seek proper help?

Could they make Vikki well enough to get her home?

What should I do?

What can I do?

What about Romy?

We were flying through the night. All around there was the strange calm you get on planes as the darkness outside descends, as lights are dimmed, as activity declines. So much normality around us. Everything quiet. Just the rush of the plane engines and the flickering images of the films on other people's screens.

And us. Trapped. Quietly scared.

If we can just get her home . . .

Several hours in I was still exhausted, unable to sleep. I was alarmed but finding it difficult to keep any focus. I slipped into a dull catatonic state. I couldn't summon the energy to be panicked. It was as if the knowledge of what was happening was already too terrifying to contemplate and my tired limbs and weary brain were shutting down for their own protection. Vikki continued to pass in and out of sleep but she wasn't getting better and I felt helpless as the hours crawled by. Stuck. Useless. And guilty. Why didn't I foresee this? Why did I let her even get on the plane? Why didn't we just stay in Melbourne?

As we approached Hong Kong, Vikki felt faint again. I called for the stewards, who gave her oxygen, which provided some relief. I held her tightly and massaged her neck once more. I was still trying to sound like a normal dad to Romy as I woke her gently and organised her breakfast, saying that

Mummy was just getting some help from the stewardesses and we would be landing soon where it would all be better. As I spoke I kept looking at Vikki's face to try to find something there, some comfort, something to reassure me that she was going to be okay. Once, her eyes met mine and she gave me a half-smile but I saw the effort it took.

As we landed, the stewards gave her oxygen again, but that time it was no help at all, and as people filed past on their way off the plane, she was too weak to stand. We sent for a wheelchair.

She was taken off the plane and a doctor was summoned but I noticed her expression had changed. Her eyes were suddenly wild and black, and her speech was full of confusion and panic. She had gone right down to a place where I couldn't reach her. To a place no one could reach her.

Suddenly her head lolled forward.

FORGET THE DOCTOR! WE NEED AN AMBULANCE! NOW! AS QUICKLY AS YOU CAN!

The airport staff registered the panic in my voice. They looked at Vikki slumped in the chair and were suddenly yelling instructions into their walkie-talkies.

Everything speeded up. All around people were pointing with urgent gestures, flinging their arms out, showing us where we needed to run, and they were lifting Vikki out of the wheelchair and then we were all in the ambulance and the doors were slamming and we were driving off, Vikki lying on a trolley, with her eyes closed, unconscious.

Hours seem to go by. We must have left Hong Kong. I look out of the window of the ambulance again as we rumble along the highway, but there are still more tower blocks. Still grey and shabby and teeming with people.

How far are we going? What if we're somewhere in mainland China? Untraceable. Missing in some vast new city without a name. Will we ever get out? Will we ever be found? Where are we going?

Suddenly we veer off the motorway down an exit road. After two more turns the ambulance slows, then stops. The doors open. Nurses appear. There is conversation. I see we're outside a hospital and it looks like every other hospital in the world, a modern concrete building surrounded by other modern concrete buildings.

Romy and I follow the trolley into the largest of them and into a waiting area with plastic seats. At one end of the room, a woman is sitting behind a desk. She beckons me forward and says something in Chinese.

'I'm sorry, I don't understand,' I say.

'Card. Card!' She points impatiently at my pocket.

I pull out my wallet. She nods. I put a credit card into a machine. I don't know what I'm paying for I don't know why I'm paying. Somebody, help me.

Then we're through and Vikki is in a cubicle on a trolley in a treatment area that is packed with people, some behind curtains, some in wheelchairs, some in chairs, some just standing, hobbling. Something is weird about the scene. It takes me a while to grasp that everyone is quiet: that's what's weird.

Everyone.

Absolutely silent.

There is no shouting, no complaining, and no talking. No one is demanding action or taking issue or just bemoaning their lot. People are holding the hands of the sick. Relatives are comforting relatives. Friends are supporting friends. Some are on their own and clearly in agony. But no one is making a sound.

I settle Romy in one of the plastic seats at the side of the room and start pacing, trying to get the attention of the doctors as they walk past, but the harder I try, the more completely they ignore me. And now, after the first surge of adrenaline, the shock is setting in. My legs feel heavy, my mind is dull, exhausted and confused.

I start looking in Vikki's handbag for something but I don't know what that is. Is it an insurance document, a special telephone number? Time and again I look in the bag but I can't make sense of it.

'Do something,' says Romy. But it's like a cry from miles away.

Vikki is awake now, her eyes staring but not seeing. She climbs off the trolley, tube still in her arm. I catch her and she half falls to the floor. I want to cry for her. She'd be mortified if she saw this scene – if she saw herself scrabbling around on the tiles, tearing at her gown and the tube but she doesn't know any of this. She is delirious.

A doctor walks past and I snatch at his arm. I say something. I plead. I can't hear what I'm saying any more, the words seem blunt and useless but there is something in the tone of my voice that is working because he is looking intently at me. My desperation is registering.

'She's ill, very ill . . . She was sick on the plane, she fainted . . . And then during the journey she lost consciousness . . .'

The doctor calls for others. Quickly they arrive and surround her. The curtain is pulled, leaving Romy and me, sitting next to each other, exhausted, on nearby chairs.

My daughter takes my arm and presses it softly, comfortingly. 'Well done, Daddy,' she says.

Later Vikki is taken to another ward for closer examination. We are told to return in an hour after they have run some tests. Romy and I race to the hotel in the centre of Kowloon to check in. We haven't left Hong Kong after all: we've been at the Princess Margaret Hospital where all the tourists are taken.

We stop off at the airport to locate our abandoned luggage. I expect to find it has all disappeared but the suitcases are there, just sitting on the floor near an enquiries desk. A little note has been fixed to the top of one of them. It says: 'Please leave. Hospital Emergency'.

20

FALLING

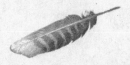

'Multiple organ failure.'

I understand what the words mean but they don't make sense. We have returned to the hospital in Hong Kong after picking up our luggage at the airport and checking in at our hotel. We are talking to a doctor outside the Intensive Care unit to which Vikki has now been admitted, just trying to understand, trying to piece it all together.

I outline how she's been battling cancer for the last few years, but they don't immediately think it's that – her deterioration has been so rapid it could well be something else: a virus, bird flu, blood poisoning, even an insect bite. They're going to monitor the situation, and they suggest that we go back to the hotel and rest. For now there is nothing more to be done. Her situation is unchanged. She is very ill but stable.

Back in the hotel room, I start the process of telling people *at home, ringing up family and friends to relay the awful news. Every time I hear their reactions I feel the shock of it all again. Like a knife cutting into me.*

'Hi. It's Carl.'

'Hi. Where are you?'

'In Hong Kong.'

'Everything okay?'

'It's Vikki.'

'What's happened?'

'She's in hospital.'

I find myself changing it so I get to the awful bit quicker. It's too much to bear to hear the cheerful initial greeting from the other end of the phone knowing the bleak news I've got to give. Now I just don't wait.

'It's Carl. Vikki's in hospital.'

After the phone calls comes the research. I'm asked by the hospital to go through old restaurant bills, receipts for wild-life parks – anything that might provide a clue as to what caused her collapse. What she ate, what she drank, what animals she came into contact with. She's too weak for them to do a biopsy but they reiterate it doesn't sound like cancer: the downward trajectory has been too dramatic.

So I'm in a race to find the answer, the right answer. I barely sleep. I send long emails to London to an old friend who is the editor of the New Scientist. *He gets in touch with the wider science community, and people I've never spoken to before send me details of possible diagnoses, which I pass on daily to the medical staff at the hospital.*

But they still don't know what is wrong with her. No one does.

Fast forward three days and it's a strange stalemate. Vikki is unconscious. Apart from the brief moment when she climbed off the trolley when first admitted, she has been unconscious throughout. She is still gravely ill but stable, and they are no nearer to finding out what caused her collapse. So we don't know how long we'll be in Hong Kong, and we find ourselves drifting through the hours, through the days, tiptoeing into the future.

The fear grows. What if she doesn't get better? What if she stays the same? What if this goes on for weeks and months? How can I best look after Romy? She's only six. And what if this just goes on and on, unchanging and with no progress? Will they ever get to the point where choices have to be made? To switch a machine off?

Please, God, no.

Vikki is in Intensive Care at the end of the corridor in a room of her own. A nurse sits two feet away from the bottom of her bed at a little desk, and spends her time taking readings from the battery of machines that Vikki is connected to – heart monitors, ventilators, blood pressure. I never see that nurse get up and walk round the room or even raise her head from either looking at the machines or writing in longhand on the charts in front of her. She must get up at some point but I never see it.

Each morning Romy and I visit, with Patricia, who has flown out to join us. Each morning we endure the same agonised anticipation as we near the end of the corridor. Will she still be there? It's a relief to hear the rhythmical sound of the ventilator going and to see the nurse seated at the end of the bed. The one thing you dread is finding the room empty.

Once there we talk to her, always talk. They tell us she can hear – hearing is the last thing to go, and sometimes as I speak I hear the bleeps on her heart monitor quicken. We always ask Romy if she wants to say anything for we are always keen to involve her, if that is what she wishes. One day she strolls up fearlessly to the bedside and starts talking to her mother in an astonishingly fluent manner about the history book she has just bought, holding it up, flicking through the pages, explaining the illustrations. It's an amazing and very touching moment to witness between a loving daughter and her stricken mum.

Mostly, though, Romy hangs back, while we take the lead, intimidated perhaps by the scene, by the sight of the bed which seems huge and forbidding, raised up as it is off the floor. Then there are all the wires and the tubes; the machines that whirr and buzz.

And there is the blood too.

One morning we go in and there is a lot of blood, more than usual. It's coming out of Vikki's mouth – a gruesome sight. Bright scarlet and bubbling up around the tube that is going into her throat. Then, as we wait down the corridor on some plastic seats while they clean her up, a woman sitting next to Romy suddenly passes out and slides onto the floor, smashing her head on the tiles so violently it sounds like someone breaking a rock with a sledgehammer.

Can it get any worse?

We comfort Romy and ask if she is okay. Her pale drawn face nods back at us but we wonder what is really going on inside her brain. What she makes of this horror. Whether she is just locking it away for a distant day in her adult future when it will all come flooding out. Wave upon wave. One jolting memory after another. There are many times when Patricia and I wonder whether Romy should be there at all but we feel on balance we should be together in this time of crisis. Most important, Romy herself wants to be with us; she has told us that on several occasions. And of course, she wants to be near her mum.

A kind offer comes through to stay with the friend of a friend who lives on Hong Kong Island across the water in the country. From our initial email exchange I somehow picture a cool, white, colonial-style mansion with house-keepers, nannies and gardeners, the essence of luxury. Home-cooked food, a chance to wash clothes, to talk, to grab some sanity.

When we get there it's a small, chaotic house hidden in scruffy woods. Some slates are missing from the roof and the walls are rough and chipped. The garden is unkempt and mostly paved with stones that have seen better days. Loosely strung wire separates it from next door's garden, which is smaller and even messier with a pair of grubby mopeds parked outside.

To get to the house you have to walk down an unlit path and across a graveyard. When we arrive there, our host warns us about the snake that pops out from time to time and nips the ankles of anyone walking along the path; the latest victim was airlifted to hospital only the previous week. There are also Komodo dragons that wander into her front room, and a pet chinchilla in a cage keeps me awake at night by racing on its wheel.

Our host writes speeches for the Chinese government and her sight is failing. She is kind and generous, but there is a sadness about her too. Her husband and adopted daughter are back in Europe, and much is unexplained about her situation here, alone, among the trees and ferns and snakes. Her husband seems happy with the separation, though she does not. I don't feel able to ask more, and months later when we're back in England, I get a sad email from her that explains it all: she has just discovered her husband has another family that he's kept secret for years.

So for the time being she lives there alone, a sweet, clever, melancholic woman, with only exotic animals and curious locals for company. Unwilling to face the awful truth of her own situation, which she seems to suspect is out there, just waiting to confront her.

We settle in and establish a grim, surreal routine. Each day we wander across the graveyard and through the forest to the roadside. We get a bus down the hill, then wait for the ferry to take us across to the other island. Once there, we get into a taxi and go to the hospital where we stop off in the little shop on the ground floor and buy our facemasks. We go upstairs, ring the bell outside Intensive Care and wait for the door to be opened. Then we wash our hands and walk through to the last cubicle on the right. After the vigil – talking to her, telling news, giving words of encouragement – we leave, always with the sharp pain of fear. Is this the last time? Wearily we return in another taxi to the ferry. Then we get the bus back up the hill. By the time we reach the bus stop at the foot of the path, it is dark. Fierce, coal-black dark. We get our torches out and, breathing heavily, walk slowly up the path as, in the background, the cicadas click and a dog barks. When we get to the graveyard, we run through it to the front door.

Over the next few days we introduce whatever normality we can into the strange, mad world we now inhabit but it gets madder. Another Englishwoman and her young daughter live in the village down the road and offer one day to look after Romy, just to give her a break while Patricia and I go to the hospital. Romy is duly taken there by the woman's housekeeper while we head off on our usual journey. When we return at the end of the day, all Romy can talk about is how the housekeeper showed her the room where she lived – which is a cupboard. Literally a cupboard.

Madder and madder.

We go to Kowloon Park one day and see a group of about a hundred pensioners doing Tai Chi in perfect

*harmony. Then we come across a beggar lying on a bed of
nails to raise funds. We see hawkers in the streets offering
colourful parrots for sale, stilt-walkers, jugglers and old
soothsayers on the shoreline. And everywhere there are
people and garish neon signs, noise, cooking smells and, in
the background, a constant low-level drilling as more
skyscrapers are built in this land of skyscrapers – the whole
city changing, moving, reinventing itself; the landscape is
a surreal film-set with us wandering round it, dazed and
lost.*

*Ten days after Vikki's admission, we're in Intensive Care at
our bedside vigil when a doctor asks to talk to us. We are
taken to a small room at the other end of the corridor.*

*'We have finally managed to do a biopsy,' says the
doctor, as she closes the door behind her and sits down.
Her voice is solemn and she fixes us with a grave,
unblinking stare.*

It's cancer, after all.

*She shows us a scan. 'The black areas are . . .' She trails
off.*

We know what the black areas are.

*'As you can see, it is everywhere. In her lungs, in her liver.
I don't know how she has survived this long,' she says.
'Remarkable.'*

'She is a remarkable person,' I say.

'She didn't know about this?' the doctor asks.

'No, she didn't,' I explain. 'She didn't want to. She didn't

want to have loads of scans. She knew that if the cancer came back, that would be it, so why go looking for it?'

The doctor nods gently.

My throat is so tight it's strangling me.

'We can see if we can get her well enough to travel in an air ambulance. To get her home in time,' the doctor says.

'Get her home,' I repeat. 'Yes. That's important.'

But two days later she isn't any better. She's worse.

Now I have to tell my six-year-old daughter that her mother is going to die. I have discussed it with Patricia. We both know it is the right thing to do. The only thing to do. Neither of us want Romy to be surprised when it happens. Or misunderstand. We don't want her to feel shut out for some reason, not privy to some terrible adult secret. We don't want her to be shielded, then have to come upon the truth accidentally or after everyone else. We want her to know. We want her to be clear so she can face this terrible news with the rest of us. So she can start to try to come to terms with it, however slowly.

'I wanted to say something to you. You know Mummy is very ill?'

In the privacy of the hotel room, I kneel unsteadily in front of my daughter. I can feel my left leg shaking as it rests on the carpet.

'Yes,' she replies warily.

'And we were hoping that the doctors could help her get better?'

'Yes.'

'Well, I'm afraid they can't.' There is a pause. My throat is raw. 'And I'm afraid that . . . she's going to die soon. I'm so sorry.'

There is a pause. For a second I see Romy struggle to take it in, the enormity of it, emotions spread-eagled across her face. Then the realisation seems to hit. She puckers up in agony, rushes towards me and flings herself into my arms, crying.

I hold her so tight I can feel her little heart thumping against her ribcage.

'I'm sorry, darling. I'm so sorry,' I say.

How do you ever say goodbye? How do you ever find the words? No one teaches you that. They can't. It's too huge. Beyond language. How do you sum it up? How do you say it all? How do you thank her?

The doctors have told us Vikki is weakening and advise us to say our goodbyes. So we each have time with her. For me, it's a blur. Like walking through a cloud. I'm reaching for sense, meaning, but everything seems foggy and blunt, and the further I reach for what I want to say, the further away it seems to drift, useless, disconnected. Inadequate. And then I'm suddenly overwhelmed by emotion, utterly swept away by tears and great cracking, moaning sobs that pull and tear at me till my ribs feel as if they're splitting and my whole body is being prised apart.

Yet somehow, in the midst of this maelstrom, in the midst

of all the clashing, roaring, emotional turmoil, I chance on something, a moment of clarity, when everything else seems to stop, as if someone has frozen the world and everything in it, apart from the two of us. And I'm able to halt the tears, get my breath and speak some simple, meaningful words. And at that last precious moment, I know, I just know, that my beautiful wife, in the midst of all her pain and anguish, in the very last hours of her letting go, can hear every one of them.

That night at the hotel, we go to bed early, checking that all the phones are working. The hospital has told us they'll be in touch if she deteriorates further, if they sense she's slipping away. Outside, the constant drilling noise that fills the Hong Kong air still hammers away in the background. There is a thunderstorm and the rain lashes the pavement. Hard and unforgiving.

I awake with a start, as if someone has shaken me. It's around four o'clock and very still, the atmosphere heavy and dank after the rain.

The sensation is startling and violent, as if, through the suffocating air, through the muffled traffic noise, someone has reached out and grabbed hold of me as they are falling.

Half an hour later we get the call and rush to the hospital.

By the time we get there, she has died.

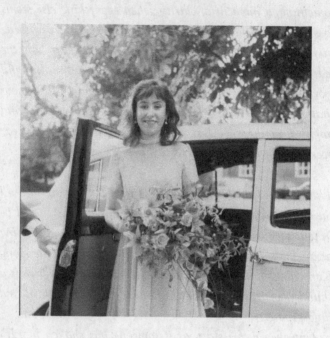

21

CARDBOARD MUMMY

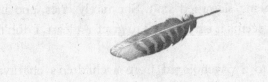

'I want to make Mummy,' says Romy, one morning.

'Erm, okay.' I haven't heard this one before.

'Can we make Mummy?' she persists.

'Er . . . well . . . the thing is, we can't actually "make" her.'

'Yes, we can,' she says. 'From cardboard!'

It is nine months since her mother's death and I have worried about my daughter. She is a quiet, self-contained child and has carried on as normal – ballet classes, riding ponies, friends coming for tea and Disney shows. I have wondered if, underneath, a deep reservoir of unexpressed grief is just waiting to erupt one day, like a geyser.

I've tried to involve her in the various rituals of grief. She helped to choose the dress her mum was buried in; she picked a song for the funeral; old photos cover her bedroom walls.

But still . . .

She doesn't talk much about how she feels, not even inarticulately, and when I raise the subject and offer her the chance to talk to someone else, someone professional maybe, she changes the subject immediately and I feel a door is being slammed shut. She rarely cries, and if she does, it seems it isn't related to grief. At least, I don't think it is.

I speak to a psychologist from a children's charity, who tells me that a young person's grief is highly unpredictable. There will be times when they want to express it and others when they do not. And there is no knowing when that might be or, indeed, how. Some children spend years keeping things buried deep inside, then suddenly open up. For others it's a gradual drip-drip of emotion. The advice is to keep talking and stay receptive. To do everything and anything they ask in expressing their grief, however weird, or unexpected it might seem at the time.

So, we build a Mummy out of cardboard.

The head is a small box, just an ordinary one from the local supermarket. This sits on a much larger cardboard container that forms the torso. At the sides, for arms, we attach two of those long cylinders that you carry posters in, along with two more for the legs. Romy draws on a face – eyes, ears, nose and mouth – and spends the most time on a highly ornate necklace, with a yellow felt-tip pen. A conservative jacket is drawn on the front with blue buttons, and lipstick is applied to the mouth, which is a slit cut with a bread knife. She is not just a Mummy made from cardboard, she is christened Cardboard Mummy.

Cardboard Mummy becomes part of the family. She sits on the sofa while we watch television. She's brought into the kitchen at mealtimes where an extra place is laid for her. At night I carry her up the stairs so she can watch over my daughter in bed, then fall asleep herself. When the weather improves and we're playing outside, Cardboard Mummy perches on a garden table.

Romy talks to Cardboard Mummy about school friends, holidays, which Disney Princess is her favourite and why. She asks her advice about clothes and brushing her hair, and in turn Cardboard Mummy is given daughterly advice and sometimes scolded. At night, before bedtime, we read fairy tales to Cardboard Mummy, and Romy kisses her goodnight.

I'm pleased about this, encouraged. Romy is engaging with something, though I'm not sure what. But something is happening. Something is moving. Something is being expressed. Instinctively I feel it's a good thing and as someone who has been worried about her emotions being locked away, I'm relieved. Thoughts and feelings are finding a voice. For that I'm grateful.

Then one day Romy asks me a question: 'Can Cardboard Mummy come with us when we go out?'

I swallow hard. 'Where do you mean?'

'In the car. When we go shopping.'

'Er . . . okay . . . Let me think about it.'

'Please, Daddy!'

Now I feel uncomfortable. Cardboard Mummy at home is one thing, but Cardboard Mummy in public? That's a different matter. Romy's relationship with her is special and private. True, some of her friends have met Cardboard Mummy when they've come round, but it has been on her terms, under her rules. Out in public it will be different, harsher – I can just hear the cries, the comments, the quips. I can see the pointed fingers, the uncomprehending looks, the questions, however genuine and well intentioned.

'*Pleeeaaaase.*'

I'm worried about the effect on Romy if I say yes.

I don't want her to be alienated or isolated, seen as the kooky kid, the weirdo who carries round a cardboard effigy, as if she's in a scene from a Hitchcock movie.

'*Pleeeeease*, Daddy.'

If I'm honest, too, I'm a bit embarrassed myself. I don't want to be seen as the kooky dad, with the kooky kid, a crackpot, a fool, the irresponsible parent who has let his own daughter spiral off into self-indulgent fantasy and whimsy when he should be helping her stay in the real world.

'DADDY, I WANT TO TAKE HER OUT!'

I strap Cardboard Mummy into the car. She sits on the front passenger seat next to the driver and fits perfectly even with the belt on. She doesn't actually come into the supermarket with us, she stays in the car – but that's only because Cardboard Mummy won't fit into the toddler's seat at the front of the shopping trolley.

We leave the car and her, then return with our shopping a bit later. I'm surprised by how easy all this seems.

It becomes a regular occurrence and I quickly get used to having this cardboard person next to me. A couple of times I stop at traffic lights and find myself getting strange looks from people in other cars. Once, in the garage, a passer-by just stops and smiles. So far, so good. It feels like harmless eccentricity. No complications. No blame.

Our privacy still feels protected. Cardboard Mummy remains, mainly for practical reasons, safe inside the car. Like some elderly relative with limited mobility, she stays put while we go about our business then return to her, with an Eccles cake or a Mars Bar, of course. Otherwise she'd feel left out. Those who see her, and no one we know does, don't get too involved.

Then one day I'm picking up Romy from her friend's party.

I head into town and Cardboard Mummy is in the front passenger seat next to me as I arrive at the venue, a semi-detached house on a street lined with trees and hedges. I want to keep the car out of the way as I'm still a little wary of being seen with my cardboard passenger, so I park on the road some distance further on, get out and walk back to the house.

I cluster around the open front door with the other parents as the party draws to a close. There is a hubbub from the living room, then a crowd of children bursts out into the hallway, laughing, shouting and sucking sweets. I immediately recognise Romy at the back of the group and she sees me too. She waves at me and weaves her way through the crowd.

'They all want to see Cardboard Mummy!' she yells, jumping up and down with excitement.

And before I have time to react, she spots the car and races past me followed by a gaggle of excited, chatting girls. I hurry after them, trying not to look too flustered. But inside I'm panicking. Help. No. Please. This is exactly what I wanted to avoid. A sort of wild feeding frenzy with Cardboard Mummy at the centre, being pawed and poked by a bunch of noisy kids. Someone will inevitably say something careless and hurtful, and Romy will be upset, parents will get involved and find it alarming, and I won't have the chance to explain clearly that Cardboard Mummy is a good idea and not a step along the road to insanity.

When I get to the car, the children are already pointing through the window at the figure in the front seat and my daughter is bouncing up and down. 'Daddy, unlock the door. Quick!'

I feebly attempt to put them off the scent. 'You can see her through the window, surely.'

'*Open iiiiit!*' screams Romy.

'*Yeeeeeaaah!*' scream the other girls.

I unlock the door and Romy makes an emphatic sweeping gesture with her hand. 'This,' she says, with enormous pride, 'is Cardboard Mummy.' And Cardboard Mummy is lifted up out of the car. I wince as numerous pairs of hands all try to get a hug with her, and she is inevitably bashed and boffed around as the girls compete to stroke her hair and be the next in line to give her a hug.

'So this is the Cardboard Mummy we've been hearing about?' One of the girls' mothers has appeared at my side.

'Absolutely.' I try to sound relaxed but I'm not feeling it. 'Travels with us everywhere. Part of the family.' I feel my cheeks go red and hot.

And then I look at the other parent and try to communicate with my eyes the way adults do when there are children around that it's okay, *really*, and it's not weird, it is in fact healthy that my daughter has made a cardboard effigy of her recently dead mother, but I see from the woman's expression, the frozen smile, the raised eyebrows and dry, forced laugh that she isn't quite convinced.

'Hmm, *lovely*,' she says, and backs away from me, ever so slightly.

I make a mental note that somehow I have to curtail this particular project now because it's all getting out of hand, and I start inventing scenarios to keep

Cardboard Mummy at home or, in my most desperate moments, to get her to recycling and out of the frame altogether. I cling to the hope that if I do this Romy will move on quickly, as they do at that age, especially if I spend a lot of money on Disney merchandise. But I know this will be a delicate and difficult thing to pull off and I don't yet have a clue how to approach it, and part of me, the socially embarrassed self-conscious part, curses the day I agreed to make a Mummy out of cardboard.

Fast forward to the following week, and before I've had a chance to sort out an exit strategy, I'm in the school playground, waiting to pick up, when a teacher approaches me. 'Romy mentioned that she wanted to bring Cardboard Mummy into school for Show and Tell. Would that be okay with you?'

'Really? Well . . . I . . . er . . .'

'We'd look after her, of course.'

'I . . . er . . .'

'I think it would be really good for Romy and all the other children.'

'Well . . . I . . .' Caught on the hop, I'm stuck. Worried about agreeing to all this but unable to come up with a reason why not. All I have is a vague hope that my doubtful tone will put her off.

'That's great, then. Look forward to it. Thanks!' The teacher claps her hands and moves off.

So I take Cardboard Mummy into school with Romy

later that week and, as I carry her in, several parents give me strange looks and I overhear one of them audibly whisper, 'Oh, *that*'s it.'

I'm filled with a sense of gloom and doom. And I worry all day and wonder how it's gone. If the party was a nightmare scenario, at least they were all her friends. At a school Show and Tell, she will be exposed to everyone. *Everyone*. Even boys. Boys! They can be brutal at that age anyway, and she has some particularly tricky ones in her class. Boys who break things and fight constantly and shout and leer. I saw one boy the other week trying to kung fu a tree. How are they going to deal with the cardboard manifestation of my daughter's bereavement? Why did I agree to it in the first place? I should have been firmer with her teacher. Why am I so bloody soft with everyone? I should have foreseen that something like this would eventually spiral out of control. Why? Why? On and on. I find myself wallowing in the brutal fire of self-reproach – the comfort blanket of the bereaved.

At the end of the day, I wait nervously in the school playground, deliberately apart from the other parents, not wanting to get involved in their conversations lest they confirm my worst suspicions.

The bell goes and the kids come out. I look anxiously for my daughter but it's the teacher who emerges first. And the teacher looks serious. Really serious. She scans the line of waiting parents and I'm utterly convinced it's gone badly. I have visions of my daughter in tears and shaking, Cardboard Mummy with a big chunk taken out of her arm by one of the brutal boys who has taken it home to hang over the fireplace, like a hunting trophy.

Oh God. What's happened?

But then the teacher sees me and her face breaks out into a beaming smile. 'She did so well. *So* well!'

And she tells me how Romy got up in front of everyone and settled Cardboard Mummy on a table, then told her class all about her: about her mummy's illness and everything that happened in Hong Kong and how we came back and how she, my daughter, chose a song for the funeral and the dress her mummy was to be buried in and how Mummy is in the ground at the church now and how we are all so sad and how we will always be sad. All the things I worried that she had never said and maybe never thought. The things that I feared were buried deep, deep down and lost forever.

And as the teacher tells me this, I feel the tears burn the corner of my eyes.

After that day Romy doesn't ask to bring Cardboard Mummy out of the house much, if at all. Instead she just sits Cardboard Mummy on the chair next to the little table where the phone lives, in our hall. She doesn't feel the need to pick her up much either. She's happy just to acknowledge her, wave at her. It's almost as if Cardboard Mummy has done her job and their relationship has changed. Romy has moved on, like a teenager who has found her independence.

Soon, Cardboard Mummy shows the tell-tale signs of ageing. One of her arms comes off when I try to move her so I can pick up the phone, and has to be stuck back again with gaffer tape. One of the cardboard tubes that makes up one of her legs starts to unravel and hangs limply at her side. There is a rip in the torso where Cardboard Mummy got bashed as I lifted her out of the car on one of her final outings.

After a couple of months I ask if Cardboard Mummy can be moved up to the attic, and Romy agrees without hesitation.

Cardboard Mummy is still there. Romy doesn't ask to bring her down at all. However, she likes to know she is safe.

From time to time we reminisce about Cardboard Mummy, about the time she came with us to the supermarket, watched the TV and ate our meals with us. Cardboard Mummy is spoken of with fondness and nostalgia, now more like an old friend who has moved away to the other side of the world. There is no question of getting rid of Cardboard Mummy, of letting that relationship go completely, no matter that she drifts further away from us as the months and years go by.

I can see her living in the attic for ever, and if we move, she will definitely come too.

And that feels right. For all of us.

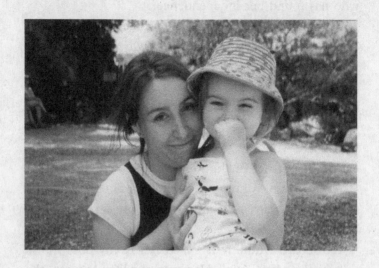

22

PRAGUE

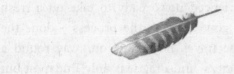

I'm standing at Gatwick airport nearly a year after Vikki's death. Romy and I are off on our travels again. But this time it isn't Hungary. This time it's different. This time there will be no friends at the other end to meet us, no cars sent to pick us up, no arranged meals, no presents, no guided tours. It's the first journey we make abroad, just the two of us, on our own. Our first proper holiday together.

It's something I feel we must do. We must keep pushing forward. Keep being active. Keep trying to make the most of life. That's what Vikki would have wanted. And in that first year when I'm lost, confused and looking for direction and reassurance, that's always the first question I ask, the question that drives me on. Is it what Vikki would have wanted?

Our destination is to be Prague, where Vikki and I

went together many times. It is where part of her family is from and is relatively close – only a couple of hours by plane. I am fairly confident. After all we've already been away and stayed with Gordon in the Hungarian capital and this feels like the logical next step. We're toughened, experienced now, ready to take on a fresh challenge. We've gone through the process – done the airports, done the travel, negotiated our way round a major European city – and Prague is only Budapest but a bit to the left. How hard can it be for a widower and his young daughter abroad?

So on a cold March day we're sitting in the departure lounge at Gatwick airport, on time, present, correct, legitimate, approved. I have managed to get us there through security with our luggage, passports and feverish worry that I've forgotten something – to turn off the gas at home or lock the door or bring the tickets. Now the first gorgeous sips of comforting coffee are burnishing my throat as I'm able for the first time to look forward and contemplate what lies ahead. I start to feel the first tiny inkling of relaxation as my shoulders drop just a little and the taut muscles around my jaw slacken, and I glance at the other travellers with a seeming air of nonchalance – and, at that very moment, I have my first crisis.

One I hadn't anticipated. Not a personal health issue or a lost wallet. I haven't forgotten to switch off something at home and it's not a sudden fear of flying brought on by some post-traumatic stress condition.

Romy wants to go to the loo.

She wants to go to the loo and I cannot take her to the Gents because I feel instinctively that she is too old for that and there are no parent-and-child loos. I can't take her to the Ladies because I'm a man, so I'm stuck.

'Daddy, I really, really, really need to go to the loo.'

Romy is insistent and I know it's important because she normally has the bladder of a camel. Briefly my mind goes back to my own little nightmare all those years ago in a toy shop in Brighton. I can feel my back tighten and invisible hands grip my throat. I lead her quickly to the Ladies and give her very explicit instructions about using the cubicles. I tell her I'll wait outside till she finishes, just by the door or as close as the other women who are going in and out will allow me without feeling the urge to get security involved.

Time passes. I wait. Other women come and go. I start to worry. What happens if Romy has fallen down the pan or can't open the cubicle door to get out?

And all my anxieties about being in charge of her for the first time away on our own, in unfamiliar surroundings, the pressure of being without her mum, our guide, chief organiser and practical person, come crashing in. Instead of reacting calmly and logically I start to panic. I'm overwhelmed by a kind of frenzied widower anxiety that blows every issue way out of proportion, sees appalling danger in the most humdrum situation and can no longer grasp proportion or perspective but just lurches from one adrenaline-fuelled moment to the next. So I find myself raising my voice, quite considerably, and yelling through the door of the Ladies that I have pushed ajar with my foot.

'DID YOU USE THE SEAT AS I SAID?'

And I can hear the ridiculous panic in my own voice, though I can't stop it. Real fear, as if I'm asking whether she has remembered her facemask during a gas attack.

A middle-aged woman emerges and looks at me suspiciously. In my befuddled state I don't even think to ask for her help.

More time passes.

'ROMY, HAVE YOU FINISHED?'

My mind flashes up all kinds of wild images. I see her clawing helplessly at the back of a locked door, tears streaming down her face, or sucked into a loo that is too big, unable to reach the door handle to lever herself back up, so shocked and distraught she can't even cry out for help. Then I picture a worse scenario, an open window, the kind that always leads out from a cubicle in a film, and Romy disappearing through it, trying to get out, only to find herself lost in some vast storeroom beyond, from which she can neither escape nor raise the alarm.

I grab the next woman who emerges by the arm. It is an ungainly move – there is an element of pouncing about it. 'Is the little girl in the cubicle all right?' I ask.

'I'm sorry?' she says, alarmed.

'She's my daughter.'

The woman relaxes but only a little. 'Well, to be honest, I didn't really see anyone,' she says.

I make a move, thinking I'll have to go in, but at that very moment Romy walks out. 'Hello, Daddy,' she says, with a sweet smile, totally oblivious.

The woman walks away and I hug my daughter, who is a little taken aback by how ferociously she is being squeezed when all she has done is go to the loo but I don't care. All I can feel is the relief that floods through me as all my anxiety and fear over being in sole charge of her just ebbs away. My heart stops pounding. My breathing slows and the blood stops racing through my veins as if it wants to blow a hole in them.

It's all right. I can cope without Vikki.

I'm not going to make a terrible mistake.

It's all right. It's fine.

I can be calm again.

Calm. Relax, breathe and—

Christ. Now I need to go to the loo myself.

Another problem. Another nightmare. The pounding in my chest returns and, with it, the anxiety. What do I do with Romy now? I scan the waiting area for anyone I could ask to keep an eye on her while I dash into the Gents. Has to be a woman, of course. I look for a kindly face. Bit of experience. A mother with kids. That would be good. Hang on, though. What about the other children? Might be a bit of bullying when my back's turned. Scrap that. Other children are an issue. I maybe need a grandma-type instead. Soft features, smiling, glasses. Vulnerable but in a good way. Stick or Zimmer frame. If they can't move it's a bonus because they can't run away with her. Hang on – that means they can't give chase if someone tries to nick my daughter. No, someone with mobility is good.

Eventually I see a likely candidate and half start towards her but then I change my mind and freeze. She might not be what she seems. She might be a decoy. Or part of a child-snatching gang. My mind is working overtime.

Just then I catch sight of a kiosk a few yards to one side. A middle-aged woman is having a laugh while serving a customer at a till. That's the answer. A kiosk: nice and public, and the woman is employed there so she's safe.

By this time my bladder is the size of a small car. 'Excuse me, can I leave this child with you?'

The woman looks confused, borderline alarmed.

'I'm her dad. I have to go to the loo. Here's my passport.'

She smiles. 'Okay. No problem.'

I race into the Gents, like a maniac, have the fastest, most uncomfortable pee I have ever had and run out again. When I return, breathless and red-faced, I see my daughter standing by the kiosk, happily chatting away to the woman at the till.

All this and we haven't even taken off yet.

The rest of the holiday is just as tiring. Being out there alone with Romy, solely responsible for getting her around, keeping her happy, warm and fed, feels exhausting. Each day I have a trip organised, meals too – I have printed out an itinerary, planned it right down to the last minute, not only because I'm terrified of screwing up but, of course, it's what Vikki would have done.

We stay at the Intercontinental – Vikki and I had gone there in the early nineties just after the revolution when it was the only place you could get a decent meal. Then the place had been packed for Sunday brunch, an all-you-can-eat affair. There was a queue that went out of the door which we joined, next to the visiting Harlem Globetrotters basketball team, who just looked bemused.

The hotel hasn't changed much – not that we'd notice: we're barely there. We go out early in the morning and come back late in the day because I'm so determined to make the trip interesting, stimulating and fun. We go ice skating in the cavernous wooden bowl of a stadium, watch elephants at the zoo, take a horse-drawn carriage trip around Prague, get cheap concert tickets to the ballet, visit a puppet museum, and walk and walk, and chat and chat, and take pictures on the Charles Bridge.

Each night after a meal we return to the hotel and spend the rest of the evening building a den by turning the room upside down. We take the sheets off the beds and the covers off the duvets and stretch them over the chairs and make little rooms – a bathroom kitted out with all the contents of our own hotel bathroom and a living room lit by the lamps we've taken off the tables next to the beds.

Eventually Romy gets tired and we collapse the den and remake the beds. While she is snoozing I read my book, which is a biography of Frank Sinatra written by his valet George Jacobs. Over forty years Jacobs did everything for Sinatra – cooked and cleaned, made his travel arrangements, bought presents for his women and children. I wish I had George Jacobs.

The days fly past and no sooner have we arrived than we're leaving. On the way out to the airport in the taxi I'm so tired I can barely move. Since Vikki died, I've felt tired pretty much all the time. But then I remember how often I felt tired in the years before, ever since she was diagnosed. Am I going to be tired for the rest of my life? At the moment it feels that way.

I close my eyes and think of the packed holiday, the sheer overwhelming tumble of sights and sounds, colours and smells. One particular image comes to mind. It's from the previous Tuesday, when Romy and I visited Prague zoo. We're on a chairlift that takes us up the hill from one part of the site to another, towards the big tortoises and the gorilla pavilion. As we ascend, I just happen to look back and see, through the clear but chilly Prague morning, the famous Dukla Prague football ground rising up through the houses on the horizon. It is a startling moment because, not only had I completely forgotten it was there, it brings with it a host of vivid memories that, combined with my surprise, seem to explode in my head. In an instant, words, images and feelings are racing around my brain, and I'm transported as surely as if I were in a time machine right back to another life.

We went there, Vikki and I, on our first trip to the city in 1990, shortly after the Velvet Uprising, the only foreigners in a crowd of 400. The club used to have crowds of 40,000 pre-revolution when it was the Communist team. That day, we sat alone, just the two of us, in the most expensive stand (it only cost fifty-pence each) and watched the fabled Dukla play in the ice and snow. It was an entertaining game in the bitterest cold – we had to keep getting up and jumping around every few minutes to stop ourselves freezing to the seats. After the game we walked round the other side of the ground and bought the entire souvenir shop, which consisted of one man with a fold-out table selling two mugs, three pennants, various posters and a couple of hat badges. It cost us less than a fiver.

The ground I had visited then was now unrecognisable – even at a distance, across from the zoo, through the houses. It looked smarter and freshly painted. Shiny and new. Things had clearly changed since the rickety old Communist days. Apparently there is a new Dukla now, the product of a merger between two other teams. The club is evolving, reinventing itself. It has a new outlook, a new reputation, a new identity. The old Dukla is no longer here. And neither is the woman who sat next to me all those years ago, laughing and clutching at my arm. That cold, splendid day is just a memory now.

As I sit back in the taxi, I look at Romy, who is dozing next to me. I cradle her head towards me and let her fall asleep on my shoulder. I gaze at the trees that rush by on the side of the road and the bright fields that lie beyond.

As the airport approaches I think of the newly minted stadium and the last few packed, colourful, demanding days. And I can't help but feel a brief glow of satisfaction. It has been exhausting, testing and emotionally trying, but it has been worth it.

For we've done it, the two of us. Just like Dukla Prague, we've found a new beginning.

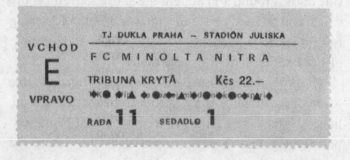

23

A DINNER DATE

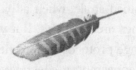

'Dinner – very relaxed. *Very* relaxed,' announces a friend of mine.

It's time – or, rather, other people have decided it's time – for me to come out of my shell, to be reintroduced to society, like a prisoner ready to be reintegrated into the outside world. I have served my sentence in the penitentiary of widowhood and now I am due for a bit of day release. Nothing too strenuous to start with. It has to be the right thing. I'm not going to be flung back into the fray. But it's time.

It's not as if I haven't had invites before. On the contrary, the last few months have been busy and I've been to various parties, but this is different. This feels more ambitious. A bigger step into a wider world. This isn't just a sympathy 'Don't leave Carl out, we'd better include him, he shouldn't be on his own' sort of invite. I've had a few of the latter, which were nice in their own way but tricky after a while because they meant I was still seen very much as the Widower. You see people wondering whether they should ask how you're getting on, and if they do, you feel duty-bound to tell them you're 'surviving' or 'managing', with a sort of pained smile, when all you want to say is that, actually, things are a bit shit. But you can't because there's still a strange protocol of politeness, a very British need to maintain appearances, cheeriness, a stiff upper lip.

But this occasion is different. I feel as if I'm being invited on my own merits, as a normal human being. It's a gathering at some friends' large detached farmhouse near Dereham. They have been especially kind to me and I feel comfortable that this first proper reintegration is in their hands. They know my situation. They know me. They've been with me every inch of the way. I can trust them.

At the back of the house there is a beautiful walled garden. They have set up a marquee there where we will eat. As I arrive, I happen to glance at the seating plan as I enter the garden. It's been stuck to an expensive piece of card and set on a large ornamental stand. So much for '*very* relaxed'.

When I look at it, I realise there are equal numbers of men and women, which means that the woman I'm sitting next to has come on her own. Of course, maybe there's a reason for this. Maybe she had to leave her partner at home, or maybe they are away on business, visiting a sick relative or unwell themselves.

Or maybe she's single. Like me.

Now my palms are sweaty and I'm faintly alarmed. And faintly excited. I wasn't quite expecting this. I hadn't prepared for it. The idea I might meet *someone new*.

This is the first time since Vikki's death that I've had to consider such a thing seriously. I feel a flutter in my stomach and my chest tightens. I look around the garden where the guests are having a drink and try to decipher who is who. I see a number of women I know who are clearly with husbands. There's a couple of other disparate groups of men and women I don't know, with a couple of other women who may be on their own. Or not. *Maybe there are several single women.* One is a fairly short woman, who already looks a little bored. The other is very thin, pinched and pale: she is holding forth and shrieking with laughter at her own jokes. And then there is a blonde in a group with two other men, who are soon joined by their wives (at least I think they're the wives). She seems to be very cool and stylish, neither shrieking nor bored. What's more, she doesn't appear to be attached to anyone.

Being an optimist and a dreamer, some would say a hopeless fantasist, I convince myself the gorgeous blonde is the one whose name appears next to mine on the seating plan and briefly imagine our evening together – an intense, fulfilling yet occasionally hilarious conversation, mostly when I make her laugh, of course, and she reveals how sad it is being alone with her enormous country pile and how she's looking for someone to share her life – preferably a comedy writer with a young daughter, recently widowed.

Suddenly I'm submerged by a wave of guilt and disgust. What am I even thinking of? Another woman? *ANOTHER WOMAN? HOW COULD YOU EVEN CONSIDER IT?*

But I just did.

Yes, but THINKING about it doesn't make you ready to DO it. It just means you're ready to THINK about doing it.

Or ready to do it.

Or ready to do it and regret it afterwards.

Or ready to do it, and then think, why did I waste so much time thinking about whether I was ready to do it when I could have been doing it a hell of a lot more?

Anyway, what do you mean do it? Do what? Meet someone? Like them? Date them? Befriend them? Snog them? Breakfast in bed? Full-on wedding in the Bahamas? Can't someone just tell me?

Ah. No. That's the thing. You will know within yourself.

How will I know?

You'll just know when the time is right.

But how will I know when the time is right?

When the time is right.

Could it be more complicated?

The call comes to go to dinner. I walk into the marquee quickly and I'm among the first to sit down. I look around as various couples come in. The blonde woman has appeared at the entrance and looks about. She glances in my direction. I watch as the thin, pinched woman comes in and walks past her. The thin, pinched woman is turning left towards me. She's walking right up to where I'm sitting . . . then past me and up the side.

Phew.

The blonde still looks around. The marquee has quickly filled up.

'If you can take your seats, please, everyone!' says the host above the hubbub.

The blonde is moving towards me. She smiles as she approaches. I smile back. She is four or five people away. She does a mock grimace as she squeezes past a portly older gentleman. She is definitely going to sit next to me now. She must be. There can be no doubt. There is no doubt. *Absolutely no doubt.* It's all falling into place.

I reach out to the empty seat on my left to pull it out ready for her to sit . . . but as I make contact, it isn't with the back of a chair but with the back of a person.

The seat is no longer empty. It has been filled by the short woman.

'Hello,' says the short woman.

'Hello,' I say, watching as the blonde keeps going and takes up a seat far away on the other side of the marquee next to a smiling young man.

The short woman glares at me for a second. There is an awkward pause, which makes me uncomfortable so

I try to get the conversation moving. 'Are you . . .
er . . . ?'

I have no idea what I'm asking but I'm rather hoping
it will just kick-start the conversation.

'Divorced,' she says, through gritted teeth, and shakes
her head.

Then she starts to speak . . .

. . . and as soon as she opens her mouth, before the
poor woman has even got to the end of her first sentence,
it hits me – like a shocking sharp blow, a bunched fist
to the jaw.

This is pointless. This is stupid.

This is impossible.

What are the chances of me ever finding someone
else – just happening to find someone else?

Three, five, ten million to one?

The very thought of it makes me want to hold up my
hands in utter defeat, throw my napkin onto the table and
walk away right there and then. The sheer impossibility
of ever finding another partner. Someone to relate to.
Someone I admire. Someone I can be daft, lazy and
difficult with. Someone I can be challenged by. Laugh
with. Rely on. Be moved by. Criticise. Praise. Love.

I realise this, all of it, in those first few seconds. And
the poor woman next to me has only had time to tell
me her ex-husband was a bit of an arse.

My heart sinks into my boots and, though I attempt to
join in with the conversation, I can hear in my dry, laboured

voice how unconvincing I am, and I can see in her reactions how obvious my negativity appears. The conversation starts to falter and she looks away. Then I look away and it's all very embarrassing, and when the first course arrives we're both so grateful for the distraction that we start eating with the desperate enthusiasm of people who have trekked across the Himalayas and not seen food for a month.

Before we've finished, I'm thinking, as she probably is, of what I'm going to do when I get to the last spoonful, whether to attempt more horribly unconvincing chat or accept the inevitable and sit in silence or even fake an illness and retire from the evening altogether. Suddenly, and mercifully, I notice out of the corner of my eye that the person on my other side is leaning back while talking to the person on *her* right, and there is an opportunity for me to join in, without looking too rude, so I gently swing round, thus detaching myself from the divorcee and fold myself into this other, different, conversation.

After a while I can sense that the divorcee has done the same to the person on her left.

And neither of us turns back for the rest of the evening.

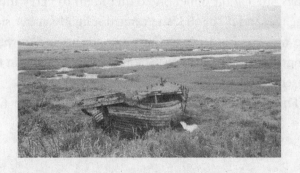

24

THE FIRST ANNIVERSARY

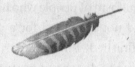

'What if there is no God and you only go round once and that's it? Well . . . don't you want to be part of the experience?'

It's the bit in *Hannah and Her Sisters* where the Woody Allen character has an epiphany about the meaning of life as he watches a Marx Brothers movie. Vikki liked that bit a lot.

Live for the moment. Live now. Enjoy it.

She didn't look to the future or the past. She didn't dream of something she couldn't have or regret other things she hadn't done. She didn't seem to carry much baggage, and if she did, she carried it lightly at her side. She was good at letting things go and moving forward, hungry for the next thing. She was good at living in the present.

The family are gathered round the TV on the first

anniversary of her death and we are watching her favourite films. *Hannah and Her Sisters* and *Sunset Boulevard*. Both stylish, funny and true. Both dry, with a cynical edge.

All very Vikki.

As we watch, it's as if she is in the room with us. Hushing her parents if one of them talks over the dialogue, despairing that it took me so long to discover William Holden. And, still, we cannot believe her absence – several times during the films I glance at the empty chair and find myself consciously counting the number of people in the room. After, when the films stop, I feel her silence, her energy gone, a gaping black hole into which our conversations disappear and our hope dissipates like mist. Without her it's still so wrong, so incomplete, so unbalanced. If she walked into the room at this minute, it wouldn't surprise me at all. It would just seem right.

There is no template for the anniversary of someone's death. There is no order of service to guide you. It's a huge event but no one tells you what to do or where to go. You're left to your own devices.

Everyone is different. I know of one person who climbs the same mountain every year to remember his wife. And another who visits the same bench in the same park in the same city because it was where he and his wife first met. Many others just let the day pass in quiet contemplation. Some, dreading the prospect, ignore it altogether.

As we gather for this first anniversary, Vikki's parents, Patricia, Romy and I, the mood is uncertain. We're wary of the huge contradiction at the heart of this particular anniversary. On the one hand it's a special day in the calendar, but on the other, it's just another in a series of days of mourning – unrelenting, unchanging by their very nature.

Even though a year has passed and we have got older, moved forward, one thing has remained achingly constant: she is still not here. Every day that fact remains the same and burns through us. Like a torch.

And so we live confusing parallel lives – the one that's here and now, the other that stopped on that fateful day a year ago, one that moves forward, one frozen in time for ever, one that embraces new experiences, one recalling a past life. Two lives that creak and groan as they rub together, like parts of a machine that don't quite fit. Exhausting, draining and sad.

In the afternoon we walk up to the graveyard. Up the hill, past the houses. It's chilly, brisk weather, with an edgy wind and dark clouds overhead. As if it has been designed for today.

We walk mostly in silence, with the odd nod to what we see around us. But I know that each of us is weighed down with a different set of voices in our heads. I find myself contemplating the things Vikki has missed in this past year – Romy singing wonderfully at school; her getting taller, more beautiful like her mother; the time we've spent with the incredibly stoical Patricia; the huge laughs we had when we all ended up playing our own version of *Strictly Come Dancing* in the living room at Christmas, me paired with Romy, the grandparents dancing with each other, my mum and Patricia as judges. We saw a wonderful production of *Mary Poppins* in London; I drew up plans to redecorate downstairs in a minimalist fashion ('It's not an art gallery!' I hear Vikki protest). Even us, today, remembering her with the films and our devotion, trudging up the hill in the stiff breeze ('Please, you don't have to. Not on my account'). She will never know these things.

Just as she will never know about the fire on the *Cutty Sark* in her beloved Greenwich; Gordon Brown becoming prime minister; the inspiring rise of Barack Obama; the terrorist attack on Glasgow airport; the demise of Tony Wilson, the one-time manager of her favourites Joy Division; the fact that the Police on their reunion tour were every bit as good as she might have imagined. She will never again experience beautiful paintings, read fantastic books, taste wonderful food.

She will never see the world grow and develop, take shape, change course. She will never again be there watching it, questioning it, pulling it apart, putting it back together. She will never again be part of the argument, and for someone so engaged, so interested, so committed to life that is another huge sadness. One of many. Far too many.

At the top of the hill, the road forks, and we go right as it sweeps round and up to the church. We're high up now and it's possible to see across ploughed fields on both sides. Only in the distance, save for one house, are there other buildings. We are increasingly isolated as we near the church, its spire creeping up out of the trees ahead.

As we turn into the graveyard I feel the brief burst of adrenaline that always accompanies a visit here, the cold shock that comes over me. A year has passed but it feels like yesterday. In one way, time has definitely moved on. Whereas Vikki's grave was the first in her row, now the whole line is almost complete with two very new graves, the tell-tale piles of freshly dug earth rising above ground level, like ancient burial mounds. One is covered with flowers and wreaths: a very recent death.

At the graveside we stand in silence. I look to the far side and see the dramatic dead tree, its bare branches reaching up to the clouds. I think of Romy clutching me a year ago as I stood on this very spot, the crowd hanging back by the graveside, her teacher, whom I had thought of as an undemonstrative woman, dabbing at tear-stained cheeks with a tissue.

Now we get out Vikki's favourite cake, Victoria sponge, and raise a glass, each taking it in turns to say a few words. I'm struck by the oddness of the occasion – the toast, the vocal tributes, a kind of birthday celebration for someone who's died. And I think of the vicar's words, which jarred a year previously – 'She's not here' – and realise how wrong he was.

She's here, all right. In that grave but also in Woody Allen's words and William Holden's screen presence, the cake we're eating and the Prosecco we're drinking; in my daughter's smile and our own bravado, our refusal to curl up and disappear on this the saddest of all days.

Never is the imprint of someone as alive as when they are dead.

Slowly, members of the family peel away and walk back across the grass to where the edge of the church-yard meets the road. I'm left alone by the grave. I stand there for a moment, thinking of nothing and everything, as the wind whistles through the nearby hedgerow.

Then I step back, pull my coat in tight, and walk away.

25

A WIDOWER'S TALE

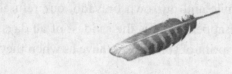

'Funny (it's what I do for a living), kind, mid-40s. Loves to dance.'

I'm poring over my *Guardian* Soul Mates entry a couple of months after the anniversary. Perhaps surprisingly, my previous dinner party experience – that sinking feeling, the impossibility of it all – hasn't put me off.

In fact, in a curious way it has encouraged me. Maybe it's my own bloody-mindedness that won't accept the odds. Maybe it's the eternal optimist that always lurks inside. But now that more than a year has passed since Vikki died I'm more ready to meet someone. Or, rather, enough of me wants to meet someone to drag the other, reluctant, person along with it. I reckon I'm always going to feel a little guilty, at least until I've taken that first step.

I've also realised that this is one of the keys to me surviving, moving on, prospering, building another life.

I don't want to live in the past, a sad, shuffling individual still in love with someone who is no longer here. I want to keep moving forward. I want to keep on living.

And in order to do that I have to accept one very simple fact.

I am not going to meet Vikki again.

I am probably not even going to meet someone *like* her.

But I am going to meet *someone*.

I have chosen this dating site above the millions of others because of its associations. There is something about the *Guardian*, with its puns and occasional literary references. It seems comfortingly twee and probably appeals to the snob in me. I always think of *Guardian* readers as sophisticated, moderate, sensible grown-ups probably because I'm a *Guardian* reader myself. Plus I don't think I'm going to meet an axe-murderess there. At worst they're going to worry about the planet too much, make their own mung bean stew, and concern themselves with the effect on their health of the vibrations from local wind turbines. Which is not the worst thing in the world. At the very least we can always be friends.

'Funny' is what I hope will appeal. 'Kind' is an attempt to say 'nice but not bland' and to suggest I'm not some monster. But 'loves to dance'? I'm not sure. I put it in because it's true and I'd also wanted to offset any suggestion that I was an old crock. I wanted to imply vitality, zest for life, *joie de vivre*. Now I just think it makes me sound gay.

There are two contrasting replies almost in seconds. One is from a woman in London who is so laid back I'm surprised she was able to summon the energy to get in touch in the first place. While sounding plausible, she isn't interested in much, apart from shopping, and my first thought is that given her lack of zip, there must be serious question marks over whether that's even true or not. I don't follow this one up.

The other lady is Polish, and also from London. She has apparently ONLY just re-joined the dating service and it was ALL because of me. And she is VERY passionate about all the things I'm interested in, plus MANY MORE and would LOVE to meet up and keeps using CAPITAL letters for emphasis, which is a bit INTENSE. In her picture she is staring into the camera with such ferocity she looks as if she's grabbed the photographer by the lapels.

I'm flattered by her interest and we have some initial exchanges that tend to follow a familiar pattern in which I say things I would like to do and she agrees enthusiastically, then adds on something else she would like to do after that, which is completely unconnected. So a typical exchange might read:

I'm interested in seeing the new Michael Frayn play at the National.

Maybe we could SALSA afterwards!!!!!

And then a couple of days later:

> I'd quite like to see the Rothko exhibition at the Tate Modern.

> Yes. And I would like to learn to ROLL SUSHI too!!!!!!

The Polish lady is enthusiastic, passionate and interested in a lot of the same things I'm interested in, but I realise, after a few days, that I'm exhausted even before we've spoken directly or met, and though intensity of the kind she possesses is often a good thing, it can also mean broken crockery and a lifetime of stress. Reluctantly, I let our contact slide and decide that maybe the whole online scene just isn't for me.

Then, about two months later, I get an email inviting me to an evening for singles in west London. It's for people in the media, which, strictly speaking, is what I am, though I detest the label, and therefore gives me at least a fighting chance of having something in common with the people there, and it's organised by a friend of a friend – so I think, what the hell? And go.

It takes place in a smart west London bar which has wooden floors, exposed brickwork and distressed chesterfield sofas scattered throughout. A shiny, successful, branded sort of place for shiny, successful, branded people.

I have prepared for this, thoroughly. I came down from Norfolk earlier that day and am staying at a hotel in Kew within taxi range. There, I sombrely consider my choice of outfit and decide on a black jacket, a blue Paul Smith shirt and pressed jeans. I'm trying to look like a relaxed, not completely obsolete middle-aged man, with a touch of experience. But when I look in the mirror, I see a pale, stressed widower with the world on his shoulders.

I don't want to be too early, and therefore suffer the awkwardness of having to get things going, so I make the mistake of arriving too late when the evening has not only got going but has virtually disappeared over the horizon. The room appears to be full of high-achieving, good-looking young people who have already managed to pair off and appear to be engaged in witty, provocative, insightful conversation. Everyone is very buff, polished, self-possessed and confident, and I feel a chill on my spine.

I force my way nervously through the throng of chatting couples, trying to look purposeful as if I know where I'm going when I'm just trying desperately to find someone on their own, and manage to steer myself into the path of a very tall woman who is coming in the opposite direction.

'Hi, I'm Carl,' I say. But my voice is dry and it comes out as 'Crrrrlll'.

'Hi, I'm Lucy,' she replies.

It turns out she's a PA for a well-known comedian and the conversation flows as she starts telling me a series of funny, informative stories about life backstage – the dramas, the pressures, the crazy fan requests. And I ask reasonable questions and we're having a proper chat. Briefly I look around and think, for a minute, that maybe I could be mistaken for one of the shiny, confident things I looked at from the bottom of the stairs as I arrived.

Then it's my turn to speak.

'What brings you here?' Lucy asks.

'I'm a widower,' I say straight away.

Now, I had anticipated this before I arrived: the big question. Why *are* you here? And I've thought through how I'll answer it, whether I will prevaricate or lie or hold back. I've decided I'll be upfront and clear with people from the outset. Get it out in the open. Stake my ground. Let people know I'm not worried about it, hoping they will then follow suit.

I have to admit, as well if I'm honest, having read one or two articles saying that the widower is a powerful, potent figure for a lot of women – vulnerable with a certain depth and emotional gravitas – that part of me, the shallow, crass part, even thinks it might be a plus.

So I smile at her after I've said it. Not cocky, just confident that I've made the right decision.

She backs away quicker than if I'd told her I had a bomb around my waist.

I hear her say something about getting another drink, but before I can react she's already out of earshot, lost in the mêlée of bright young normal non-widowed people.

I'm surprised but I don't immediately feel I've said a terrible thing. I think it's just come as a shock to her. You don't expect to meet youngish widowers anywhere, especially at a do like this. And the fact is, I'm so used to the label 'widower', because I live with it every day, that I may have misjudged the impact it could have on someone else. Someone who came out for an optimistic, fun, young, forward-looking event, has suddenly found herself in close proximity to someone who has death and bereavement oozing out of every pore. No wonder she ran for it.

I resolve not to jump in next time with the information but to hold it back. Not to lie exactly, which I'm terrible at, actually technically bad – I go bright red and stutter and stare at the floor and basically look like the last person you'd want a relationship with – but be a little less bold with it, a little less upfront. To pick my moment.

Later, after a meandering and desultory conversation with a Middle East correspondent, who keeps looking over my shoulder, I end up in a corner of the room talking to two very attractive women in their thirties who happen to know each other. We share a few laughs.

'Have you been to one of these before?'

'No,' I say. But I keep quiet about the widower stuff.

One of them, the dark-haired one, separates off, distracted by something someone says behind her, and I'm left talking to the blonde one with short hair. Gradually the talk becomes a little more personal. Less about anecdotes. About actors and showbiz connections. She starts to tell me about her disastrous former relationship in some surprising detail, and when she asks me about my last relationship I feel instinctively that the time is right because we're swapping confidences.

'My wife died just over a year ago.'

Her face freezes in an expression of astonishment and her jaw drops.

At that point, her friend, the dark-haired woman, turns back and re-enters the conversation, introducing us to two men, also in their thirties with tanned faces and amazingly white teeth. They look intently at the girls with hungry eyes, but although they say hello to me as well, they never take their eyes off the girls.

The blonde one with the short hair looks so grateful that the others have appeared she practically bursts into tears and hurriedly steers her friend and the two lads as far away from me as possible, right up to the other end of the bar.

Alone again, I find myself thinking there is clearly no time at which it's a good idea to announce that you're a widower. Forget holding it back. Forget it altogether. It's not a question of being shocked. People just don't want to know. It's too depressing. To them I'm just a ghoul. I'd be better off telling them I was a murderer – at least that's interesting, even curiously glamorous. Being a widower is just bleak. Avoid the damn subject altogether, I decide.

A few hours later and the evening is drawing to a close. Suddenly that melee of people has thinned out. Across the far side of the room some people are collecting their coats from the cloakroom at the bottom of the stairs. Most are leaving in groups. It doesn't look like many people have paired off but even the ones who are leaving on their own still look contented and self-possessed. And much happier than I feel.

I find myself one of the stragglers, uncertain of when I should go. Unwilling to leave, but with no good reason to stay, I find myself disconnected from what is left of the crowd. Finally, in a bid at least to talk to someone, I get into a conversation with one woman I already know, an actress I've worked with on several occasions, someone I'm not romantically interested in, which at this stage is something of a relief.

Just then my arm is grabbed. I turn to see the organiser, who pulls someone else towards me, an embarrassed-looking woman, about the same age as me. She is tall, dark and carrying a coat. 'This is Rachel – she's a TV producer.'

'Hello, I'm Carl,' I say.

'I need a cigarette,' she replies. 'You coming?'

We go outside and sit at a wooden table on the pavement nearest the door. A steady stream of people come

out of the bar as we're talking and I realise she's probably the last person I'll speak to that evening.

'You ever done anything like this before?' I ask, as she
puffs away.

'Oh no,' she says. 'I couldn't face the rejection.'

Interesting. Revealing. She's opened up a little to me
already.

We talk about children and careers. We have things
in common.

I mention the name of a well-known celeb.

'Oh. You know him too.'

'Saw him only the other week.' My confidence is
growing. More things in common. Even better. 'His
partner is godmother to my daughter.'

'Really?' she says. 'Nice people.'

Yes. Yes. Yes. I'm really into my stride now. At last. A
shared world. Shared views. A form of intimacy, without
going into the dangerous territory of bereavement.

'Yes, they're great, aren't they? They've been very
good to me since—'

She looks at me. 'Since?'

Shit, I shouldn't have relaxed. 'My wife – er . . .' I
stumble.

'Er . . .' I feel trapped in the headlights.

She takes another long drag on her cigarette.

'My wife, er . . .' I'm completely stuck. *What? Left me,
departed, divorced me, ran off with someone else?* The
possibilities rush through my head. I could still save

233

myself even now. But what's the point? It has to come out sooner or later. 'Died.'

There. I've said it.

I look up and expect her to go, just like the others. I expect her to see this screaming symbol of death in front of her, then bolt for the hills. But no. She's still there. Smiling. Seemingly unperturbed.

I like this woman.

Now, for the first time, I feel the confidence oozing through my veins. I feel renewed. I feel bright and optimistic. At last.

She puts out her cigarette but she's still smiling. Someone who doesn't think that death is out of bounds. Someone who is unworried by the widower opposite her. Someone who can handle my shit.

We talk more and more. We get on. We communicate. We get way beyond the death thing. And I start to think maybe, finally, just as the evening is finishing, I've met someone. Not just met someone but *met* someone. Someone I have things in common with. Someone mature and interesting and funny. Someone I can talk to honestly. Someone I can be relaxed with.

She keeps smiling at me. She must be enjoying our chat. *Surely*. She *must* be comfortable. She *must* be feeling, like me, that *possibly* there might be the *faintest* glimmer of something, a connection of some sort, *maybe*, the smallest chance *potentially*—

'It's getting late,' she says. 'I've got to go. Nice meeting you.' She smiles again, stands, then puts on her coat, leans across the table and pecks me chastely on the cheek. Then she turns and walks purposefully down the street. Within twenty yards she has flagged down a cab and got in, and I watch as it drives off into the London night.

She doesn't look back once.

And then it dawns on me that for all my obsessing about being a widower, for all my worries about where and how to make the announcement, I've completely forgotten about something else, that tiny little thing called attraction, the indefinable spark, the mysterious pull that draws people together regardless of whether either of them is bereaved or half mad.

It's clear now. For all her smiling, patience and understanding, *that* was probably the reason she walked away. *She just wasn't really interested in me.* And that's something, oddly, I hadn't previously considered. With the blindness and self-absorption of the recently widowed, it has so far been all about *me*. At the dinner party, with the short woman, it was all about *my* needs. What *I* wanted. About the difficulty of *me* finding someone else. I hadn't even considered the possibility of that person not wanting to find *me*.

I think back to adolescence, to the various knock-backs everyone receives. All of that emotional turmoil is now a part of my life again, my new life as a single man who would prefer not to be single. All of that must now be taken into consideration – the possibility of rejection, the potential for getting it wrong, for misreading signals, miscalculating the odds. The hopes dashed. The expectations not met. The inevitable let-downs.

I suddenly feel weary and resigned to the prospect of dealing with it all, on top of the grief that still hangs like a millstone around my neck. I feel shrunken, weak and fragile. Vulnerable. Ill-prepared for the harsh battering of the dating game.

And I just want to go home.

The sky is bathed in moonlight, but there's a chill in the air. I can hear one of the doors into the bar being bolted shut. I get up from my seat and head off. As I walk back along the road past the other tables and chairs on the pavement I notice the two young women I frightened off earlier that evening, the blonde and the one with dark hair. They are sitting on the knees of the two young men who couldn't take their eyes off them. The women's arms are wrapped around the men. And they are kissing them passionately.

26

ALWAYS

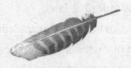

A photo of Vikki, bright and irreverent in fancy dress. Schools Dinner. Hertford College, Oxford, 1983. A lock of her hair. Her wedding ring. Copies of the orders of service from her funeral. Some perfume. A poem. A soft toy. A favourite dress. Romy is making a memory box, selecting things she can put into it.

I have been conscious for a while of wanting her to do something like this. All the bereavement literature on young people says that it helps but she's just not been ready. Or I've not been ready. Now Romy has selected things and I have just made suggestions. As has Patricia.

On the day that we do it, I find myself hanging back, finding other things to do. But Patricia steps in, as she always does, and it becomes a rather lovely girls' art project while I remain in my room, listening to them chatting as they work.

That early sense of touching Vikki's things and feeling in them an almost electric connection to her has never left me. If anything, it has got worse. I am barely able to go near her things without experiencing a crippling sense of distress, a feeling of disquiet, as if I'm disturbing some ancient fundamental law.

After an initial flurry, her things still litter the house. All her shoes are in our dressing room next to the bedroom. Her clothes are in the wardrobe. Her coats still hang in the hallway. I see them every day as I move from room to room but their mere presence doesn't disturb me. Just as long as I don't touch them. Or try to move them. Then it's as if something inside me tightens and twists.

Patricia has found the perfect memory box, a square, sturdy wooden one, which is spacious and has a flip-top lid. Together she and Romy have painted it – brightly coloured stripes, nothing mournful.

They call me when it's time to put the objects in and I emerge warily from my cocoon. It helps that they're more relaxed, more matter-of-fact about the task as they place the items carefully in the box, announcing them out loud as if to a watching audience. Then the lid is closed and the box slid carefully into its own resting place on a corner of the landing, just under the window.

At the end, Romy seems happy, content, as if a very necessary job has been completed. And as I watch her skip off down the corridor I sense that it has been an important moment for her. 'Thank you,' I say to Patricia, who seems relieved as well.

Another small step in a very long journey.

I don't want my daughter to forget her mother.

I don't want to forget her mother.

I don't want anyone to forget her mother.

We have many photos of the three of us. Vikki and I were conscious that she might not be around for ever and wanted to try and record as much as we could. They are in shiny yellow envelopes piled high on shelves on the landing, each one labelled with dates and contents. There are holidays, school events, family gatherings. Some have been put into beautiful delicate photo albums, but that job had only just started when we went on our last holiday to Australia.

We have little, however, in the way of video, but that wasn't our style, who we were. We were so obsessed with being there, being in the moment, that it was something we rarely considered. We hated other parents perpetually watching their kids through a lens. We didn't even have a video taken of our wedding.

We always believed in those still images, in the classic capture of a moment. To us, somehow, videos always seemed a bit crude and lacking in atmosphere. But now that Vikki's gone, part of me regrets the paucity of film. There are videos of Romy's birthdays and of her christening; a few holiday adventures; some Christmas and

Easter footage. But not the kind of complete library that others enjoy.

I worry for Romy. I worry that there is so much of her mum that she will never see. The way she walked. Her face as she spoke. Her beautiful expressive hands. The rocking motion of her whole body as she laughed. The motion. *Her* motion. Vikki in the act of living.

Maybe because of the lack of videotapes, I determine to bring her to life in other ways. I write an account of our last years together and tuck it away in an envelope so that Romy can read it if she wants to, at some point in the future. I print off the dozens of emails I received at the time of the funeral and place them in a special envelope in the memory box.

Increasingly, too, I also find myself consciously involving Vikki in conversations with Romy so she gets to know something of her mother – her opinions, her likes and dislikes. What she thought and felt about the world. What she valued. What she held dear. What she stood for. This is tricky, though. If I do it too much it sounds false, and Romy starts to feel she's being lectured at, too little and I worry that she will lose the sharp, defined sense of her mother that other children, who have day-to-day contact, retain. And it's difficult just to find the right moment. The moment when it feels natural, organic, unforced. Sometimes I listen to myself and hear my own awkwardness as I crowbar Mummy into the conversation in a desperate fashion, as if I'm trying to win some kind of award or fulfil a bizarre quota.

Romy: 'I want to go riding this weekend.'

Me: 'You know that Mummy liked riding?'

Romy: 'Yes. [Ignoring me] Can I wear my new jeans?'

Me: 'And, actually, she, er . . . had quite a lot of pairs of jeans as well.'

A few weeks on I finally find myself sorting through Vikki's possessions. Prompted by the memory box, I have felt the need to overcome my misgivings and just get stuck in. There's a lot of stuff to get through – she was a hoarder. There are bin-bags full of ancient holiday brochures, old plane tickets and itineraries; suitcases full of clothes; boxes of ancient Christmas cards, Valentine cards and postcards.

There are even bags in the attic full of old leaflets for local attractions – the Victorian workhouse museum at Gressenhall; the Shire Horse Centre at West Runton; the glass-blowing factory at Langham; the Thursford collection, Europe's biggest collection of Wurlitzers – all of them trips we made as a family; each shiny leaflet now its own painful retelling of her absence.

This clear out is hard but I want to do it. I feel I have to. It has been more than a year now. Life is moving forward, and if I'm frightened of moving forward with it, I'm also frightened of being left behind. I don't want to be a Miss Havisham, still tending her possessions even as they're choked by cobwebs.

Besides, there is opportunity now. Opportunity that seems to shout, '*Do* something!' Romy is settled at school and doing longer hours. There is a lull in my work, and the year of funerals, headstones, letter-writing, form-filling is over. My social life, such as it was, has taken a step back too. There have been no more emails since the singles evening in west London and I'm not unhappy about that. I imagine myself on some sort of blacklist that is currently whizzing round: 'Widower. King of bleak. Nice guy but complete downer. Please don't invite him. We've had complaints.' I wouldn't have the stomach for it anyway.

Since that first hysterical bout of action, since the Polish lady and the women who fled from me in west London, I've found myself sliding backwards, doubting I'm ready for it. Ready for anything. For even as I sort through Vikki's things, even as I try to progress, I feel as if I have ground to a halt once more – emotionally and spiritually. Even as I force myself to be busy and active I feel strangely stuck, strangely inert, no matter how furiously I strive. I'm progressing but I'm not. I'm moving forward but I'm still staying exactly where I am. I'm doing things but they still seem part of her, connected to her, somehow anchored in the past. The holiday in Prague, then sorting through her possessions, they're positive but they're all still part of a life that was. I feel as if I'm not yet making decisions by myself, just as me. And I have no idea how I do that. How I become this new person. Independent. Alone.

If denial, anger, bargaining, depression and acceptance

are the five stages of mourning, they should add on a new one which is . . . 'What the hell do I do now?'

It's so hard when you have been part of a team and the captain is suddenly gone. For that is what she was. We may have shared responsibility for everything – childcare, breadwinning, domestic duties; we may both have made valuable contributions in our different ways, but there was only ever one skipper.

And we never had that conversation. The one that people are supposed to have. 'When I'm gone . . .' It was partly through habit, for we both believed in living for the moment rather than projecting forward, and it was partly circumstance. The end, when it came crashing down, was so fast that we never had time. Yes, I spoke to her at the end in the Hong Kong hospital but it was just me saying the words.

So I find myself thinking about talking to her one last time. What it would be like. What I would sacrifice for the chance to do that too. Just once. For twenty minutes. What I would give up – an arm, a leg, a year of my life? Once. I just want to speak to her once.

'Of course you want to speak to me. I want to speak to you. But we can't. That's death, isn't it?'

'Is that you?'

'Of course it's me.'

'Are you okay?'

'Yes. Better than you by the look of it.'

'Oh my God, I miss you.'

'I miss you too.'

'This is unbelievable.'

'Keep your hair on.'

'I'm sorry – it's just I've been desperate to talk to you.'

'Me likewise.'

A beat.

'I just wanted . . . There's so much . . . I need your advice.'

'You don't.'

'I do. I do.'

'You just think you do but you don't.'

'Well, for starters . . . I've sort of started meeting other women.'

'And?'

'Is that okay?'

'Of course it is. As long as it's not some Russian lap dancer.'

'Really? Just like that? I mean, how could I ever sleep with another woman?'

'Course you can. You're a man, aren't you?'

'Yes, but what about you?'

'I'm dead. Move forward.'

'But—'

'Relax. It's only sex.'

'Really?'

'You know what I mean.'

'What about everything else? I just feel so unsure.'

'You know what to do.'

'Do I?'

'Yes. You were married to me for twelve years. You knew me for twenty-five. Of course you know what to do. You've just got to get on with it.'

'I know.'

'That's the only thing I'd be really cross about. If you didn't make the absolute most of every single day. You will do that, won't you?'

'I promise.'

'And, above all, look after our lovely daughter.'

'I will.'

'I love you always.'

'I love you always too.'

There is a pause. Then I speak once more. 'Can we chat again soon?'

'Don't be a fookin' tosser.'

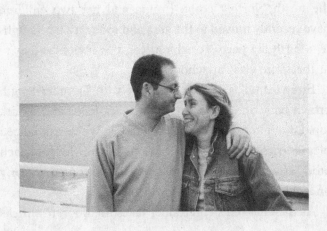

27

EMMA

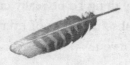

I meet her at the local village hall, on a day when I'm not trying to meet anyone. Which is probably why it happens.

It's a neat brick and flint building in an elevated position overlooking one of the small villages that pepper the north Norfolk coast. Emma and her two children have recently moved to the area and today it's her daughter's birthday party, to which Romy is invited – they're in the same class at school.

Emma is tall, slim and attractive with shoulder-length brown hair. She is wearing tight black jeans and a dark top. I don't know very much about her. We've exchanged pleasantries at pick-up time and acknowledged each other at a couple of school events, but someone, early on, told me she was a widow too.

As the children's entertainer takes the floor, to shrieks

of delight from his young audience, we find ourselves standing near each other at the back of the hall, nursing cups of tea.

Then Emma turns to me and says simply, 'How are you?' She looks at me with a clear, fearless expression and I know instantly what she's asking. How I'm coping, not with the day or the shopping or the weather, but with the whole cataclysmic business of losing my wife. And after all the baggage that other people bring to the phrase – their fears, their timidity, their wish to utter it, then run from the answer – that's such a relief to hear, it makes my heart sigh.

Almost immediately she's asking what happened in Hong Kong and I find myself able to talk about it as if we've been friends for years. We share anecdotes about grieving children, we compare notes on the arduous business of sorting out estates and commiserate about the dark days, the depression and feeling cast adrift.

Someone once wrote that the bereaved are a club, like the famous, who are only truly happy in each other's company. And I can see why. There is an immediate shorthand between us: we're able to change tack effortlessly, to follow each other, to understand. I mention a word or a phrase and she immediately picks up on it with a knowing smile. I hint at the weird, conflicting emotions I experience, and she's immediately there with me; Emma just gets it.

I'm relieved and grateful and I feel a sense of warmth, and for the first time since my wife's death, I don't feel alone, I feel companionship.

I drive away after the party in a different world, already thinking of her. Seeing her in a different light. Sitting next to her at school events. Walking down the road hand in hand. A couple. A pair. A new life. I'm even listing the advantages of pairing up with a widow. The lack of divorce angst. No lurking ex-husbands, no jealous ex-partners, no screwed-up children with divided loyalties.

A clean slate this way. Pure, no fault of ours. A fresh start. Noble. Honourable. Touching. Right. Everyone will approve. No sly digs about divorce. The old people in the village will be crying into their handkerchiefs and sobbing, 'That's so *lovely.*'

WHAT?

I catch myself mid-flow.

What are you thinking of? *WHAT?*

A relationship with another bereaved person? *Are you crazy?* What are you going to talk about with another widow? Death? Long-term illness? Bereavement benefit? Is it going to be a competition? I can out-bereave you! My suffering is greater than yours. How are you feeling today? I bet I'm worse. How many suicidal thoughts have you had today? Pah! I've had more!

And do you have anything in common apart from death?

You don't know. You barely know the woman. She might like morris dancing and Wilbur Smith. She's a widow, but that doesn't make it a good idea. It actually makes it quite a bad one.

Plus it's just too damn easy. Too convenient. Isn't it supposed to be harder than this? I, as a masochist, with my lists, manic walk, piles of paper and furious endeavour, need things to be much more difficult, don't I?

By the time I get home I've dismissed the whole idea completely, and that is how it remains for a few months. Our paths still cross while dropping off or picking up kids from school and we have friendly conversations. From time to time there is an edge of flirting too – a look, a laugh, a brush of the arm. But nothing happens.

Then one evening we both find ourselves at a young-widows' meeting – a support group set up for people under fifty who have lost a partner. It takes place at a local village, in an old-style chintzy pub dining room with a dark patterned carpet and a low Artex ceiling. It's a small room and the tables are close together. For some reason, the acoustics seem to reverberate. If you put your knife down too hard, it sounds as if someone's playing the cymbals.

It's also Saturday night and full to the brim – mostly couples. Some are quite young and eager. A few look like they're on first or early dates. There is that special keenness. One nervous chap near us keeps leaning across the table towards his partner, like a mongoose sizing up its prey. Only four of us turn up at the meeting, the first for the fledgling Norfolk branch: Emma, myself and two others. There is a man from Norwich, a shy, utterly bereft individual, and a woman of about fifty, who is one of those unreal, smiley people always looking on the positive side to the extent that she seems almost to be enjoying her grief: 'Ten years now. It's been ten years! I'll never stop talking about it!' Emma is the same wise, sensitive, fearless person I met at the party. I don't know what they make of me – I try to listen, I try to be honest, but I have to crack the odd gag as an antidote to all the grimness.

It starts like an AA meeting as we announce ourselves, and even now I can remember the illnesses – industrial accident and three types of cancer: brain, breast and ovarian – better than the names of the other people. We go round the table and swap stories.

'Was yours drawn out?'

'No. Quite quick at the end.'

'Did you go the hospice route?'

'No, she had treatment at home.'

And because we're chatty and open with one another, and it's Saturday night in a restaurant, we could be comparing notes on our holidays.

We talk about our last few years. About the onset of illness and treatment (though in the case of the accident there was no warning at all), the aftermath and how we're coping. There are lots of nods of assent.

'Still waking up with nightmares?'

'I have flashbacks.'

'Really? That's interesting.'

'Yeah, lot of blood in mine.'

'Lot of blood.'

Out of the corner of my eye I notice a couple quite near to us nod to each other quietly, get up and leave the room.

'How have your children coped?'

'One is doing very well. The other not so. They went through a phase of not eating. A lot of violent behaviour.'

'I've heard that that can be a good thing. To get it out.'

'It's hard to see that when your twelve-year-old tries to stab you with a cake fork. And my father isn't well.'

'What's wrong with him?'

Another couple leave.

'Everything really – hips, lungs, he's on dialysis three times a week.'

'Sounds tough.'

'It is. And I have to change all his dressings myself. We had some home help but that got lost in the cuts.'

'You never get over it,' says the cheerful woman, cheerfully. 'Never. I've been bereaved ten years and it feels as if I've barely begun!'

I make my excuses to go to the loo. As I get up I realise we've almost cleared the room.

Afterwards, in the car park, I run across to Emma as she's getting into her car and we share thoughts about the evening – she's surprised and pleased that it went well, though I feel I have to point out that it didn't go so well for the other diners. I tell her how thankful I was she turned up. She returns the compliment.

At the end there is a curious moment. The conversation finishes, and we're about to depart, but neither of us seems to want to bring it to a conclusion. So she stands there and I stand there and I'm suddenly aware that we're quite close together. She doesn't seem inclined to move away, and neither do I, and we both remain, not saying a word, like two boxers in a pre-fight ritual, our bodies facing each other, eyes together. Smiling rather than snarling but already somehow attached, locked together by a strange energy neither can fathom but both can feel.

Fast forward a few weeks and I've decided to invite Emma round for the evening, along with a few friends, to watch a movie. It isn't unusual, I've done it before, but the other four couples are just that, couples. Emma and I are the singles.

I'm conscious that I want her to come round but it's a vague notion beyond that. The attraction is obviously there but it's young and unformed. It hasn't coalesced into anything solid or real. In my mind I've already gone to the altar and back but in real terms I cannot translate that into anything tangible. So, I don't know what I'm asking from the evening. Certainly at its outset, I'm as focused and sure of myself as a teenage virgin – excited, terrified and vaguely hopeful. There is no plan. I just want her there.

We all share a takeaway and a few drinks, then a key moment arrives as everyone takes their places to watch the film. I go out to make teas and coffees, and when I return I notice that a space has been left for me on the sofa next to Emma. It feels like a moment of huge significance. As if everyone is already several steps ahead of me. And they've just assumed . . . Well, what have they assumed? That we're an item? That we're together?

What have *I* assumed? That we are too? I'm confused at this point because I realise I have no idea what I'm doing. I like this woman and I have invited her but on what basis? That she's a mate? That she's a mate but may become more? Christ, is this a date? I haven't been on a date for twenty-five years. What is actually going to happen?

I become incredibly self-conscious and just stand, looking around the room, airily feigning nonchalance as if I'm searching for my car keys. It's clear there is only one place I can sit but I'm too embarrassed to sit in it, so I try to make out I don't see it and glance around me on either side. If I was trying to avoid attention, this was the wrong thing to do. Everyone turns towards me. Together. With perfect timing. As one. As if a director had said: 'And TURN.'

So I'm standing at the door and everyone is looking at me. Emma, being the straightforward and honest person she is, pats the sofa next to her. 'There's a space here,' she says.

Which only makes it worse for me because it underlines how completely fake my failure to see it in the first place was. And I absolutely have to sit there now but I feel utterly paralysed and can't because everyone is staring at me, as surely as if a director had said: 'Just STARE.'

And so I stand there, for what seems like an age, leaning forward slightly in a wildly unnatural pose, as if I am testing the balls of my feet for some highly specialised medical experiment, feeling utterly trapped. I can't retreat. I can't move forward. I just have to stay rooted while a roomful of eyes bore through me and my skin burns and my neck tightens and I begin to wonder, in my desperation, if I shouldn't just fall on the floor and feign a heart attack – something, to judge from previous experience, I am obviously quite good at.

Just then, mercifully, the opening dialogue from the film kicks in, diverting everyone's attention back to the TV screen and I take the opportunity to scuttle in and sit down next to Emma. As I do so I blow out my cheeks and carelessly scan the room one final time just to show any lingering doubters that it was actually my plan all along.

I don't think they're convinced.

I don't really watch the film at all. I'm just hugely conscious of the person I'm close to. Inevitably there is some physical contact, because I'm sitting next to someone on a tightly packed sofa.

I try to relax but every time it happens I wonder. Is it deliberate? What does it mean? Our shoulders rub. Is it a sign? Her elbow brushes against mine. Is she coming on to me? Part of my leg touches part of hers. Does this mean we're an item? Every moment seems to have more meaning than the Ten Commandments.

Or maybe it's just cramp.

When the film ends, everyone gets ready to go. They pick up their coats and make for the door. As the last couple, Caroline and Jack, depart, they ask Emma whether she wants a lift home. 'Yes, please,' says Emma, and starts to put on her jacket.

But now I'm trembling because I want to talk to her. Alone. I want to test this all now. I want to know where we stand. I have to find out. 'Er . . . Just wondered . . . er . . .' I interject, without a clue as to what I'm going to say.

'I'll get the car,' says Jack.

He disappears. Caroline still lingers in the doorway. Within earshot.

'Yes?' Emma asks me.

'I just wondered if you, er . . . ?' I have to make her stay somehow. But I can't speak to her in front of other people. I look at Caroline, longing for her to walk out of earshot, but she's rooted to the spot.

'Sorry?' says Emma, clearly confused.

Caroline is looking at me now as well as Emma.

I *have* to make Emma stay. *Have* to.

'Here's Jack with the car,' says Caroline, as headlights appear.

Emma lingers, about a yard behind as if she wants me to say something, and I want to, but I'm too slow because I'm agonising about what to say and she turns back towards the door to leave. As she puts one foot on the doorstep I do the most embarrassing thing I could possibly do: I sort of lunge at her and grab her arm while asking in a squeaky voice, 'Do you want to help me with the dishes?'

'What?'

The words seem to bounce around the hallway and I'm immediately ashamed of them but now I've said them I have to repeat them. 'I was wondering if you would like to . . . to . . . er . . . help me sort out the dishes.'

Both women look bemused.

'Car's here, Emma,' says Caroline.

I can hear it revving outside as Emma stands literally half in and half out of the house, thinking. I look pleadingly at her.

'Bye, then,' Caroline says to me, and turns towards Emma.

'It's okay, I'll stay,' says Emma.

'Oh, *bye*, then,' says Caroline, kissing both of us. As she leaves, I can't help but see the faintest of smiles on her face.

Emma and I go into the living room again and I order a taxi for later. But how much later? What am I trying to do? What am I trying to ask? The teenager in me is panicking again. We make small-talk for a bit but there are only the two of us so there is nothing to hold things up any more. Nothing to prevent it coming out. And I find myself saying, 'I was . . . wondering . . . whether you . . . wanted to . . . to . . . to . . . *go out some time?*'

The words sound so strange, so alien.

But she's okay with that. She doesn't laugh or scoff. She doesn't jump in and say no. In fact I can see she's thinking it through. *She's taking it seriously.*

And it feels good. The atmosphere between us changes form, takes new shape, becomes visible. Becomes Something. It's definitely there. *Definitely.*

'I'm not sure. What if it didn't work out?' she says.

What?

What?

I hadn't considered this. Hadn't thought for a minute

she would have got there before me and planted a great big question mark against it. 'We could just try it,' I say. I'm trying to sound loose now. Casual. Take it or leave it. But it comes out defensive. 'No pressure,' I squeak, as if the amount of pressure would be the equivalent of that experienced by astronauts on re-entry.

'Maybe. I'll think about it,' she says.

'Of course. No pressure,' I reiterate.

Her taxi comes oh-so-soon and she leaves, and I feel deflated.

This isn't the dramatic conclusion I had somehow expected. No great moment after all. No big kiss. Huge embrace. No tears of joy. Not even a face slap and a rush to the door.

'"*I'll think about it,*"' I mutter to myself. 'Bloody cheek.'

But as I shut the front door behind her, and see the twin lights of the taxi suddenly blaze at the window, then quickly fade as it turns, I get the strangest feeling and my whole body fills with a sense of well-being. I think of that other first enigmatic encounter, thirty years and more ago, in the cobbled quad, the match blown out, the woman with the beautiful eyes and the way that turned out. And I have a strange sense of certainty – for the first time that evening, for the first time in months – that this is the start of something, rather than the end.

ACKNOWLEDGEMENTS

Thanks are due to my book agent Jonathan Lloyd and to my TV agents Nick Marston and Camilla Young, at Curtis Brown, for their belief and support. Thanks as well to Charlotte Hardman, my editor, for her enthusiasm and patience through many a rewrite and the rest of the team at Hodder and Stoughton - Fiona Rose, Veronique Norton and Naomi Berwin for all their hard work. This book would never have been written without early encouragement from Morwenna Banks and for that I will always be grateful. And finally, a massive thank you to my partner, family and friends who have all been so supportive to me on this journey.

The charity 'Breast Cancer Now' is the UK's largest breast cancer research charity and is dedicated to funding research into this devastating disease. Following Vikki's death I set up a tribute fund in her name. If anyone would like to donate they can do so at https://inmemory.breastcancernow.org/vikki-sipek

Facebook: @CarlGorhamAuthor
Twitter: @CarlGorham1